PHYSIOTHERAPY

IN SOME

SURGICAL CONDITIONS

JOAN E. CASH

BA, FCSP, DipTP

FABER & FABER
3 Queen Square London

First published in 1955
by Faber and Faber Limited
Second impression 1955
Second edition 1958
Third edition 1966
Reprinted 1967
Reprinted with minor revisions 1968
Fourth edition 1971
Fifth edition 1977
Printed in Great Britain by
Butler and Tanner Ltd, Frome and London
All rights reserved

ISBN 0 571 04910 9 *(hard bound edition)*
ISBN 0 571 04911 7 *(paper covers)*

© *1977 Joan E. Cash*

Foreword to First Edition

With the rapid advances that have taken place during the past ten years in anaesthesia, blood transfusion services, chemotherapy, including antibiotics, together with a better understanding of the response of the body to trauma, all surgical procedures have been rendered freer from danger or complication. At the same time, enormous progress has been made by the newer specialities of neurosurgery, plastic surgery and thoracic surgery, the latter more recently embracing several common lesions of the heart. Therapeutically, therefore, surgery has more to offer today than ever before, and physiotherapy has contributed greatly to these exciting developments. It has evolved special pre- and postoperative treatments and exercises, not only for these new procedures, but also for the more orthodox type of operation, and in these latter has minimized the risks of postoperative chest complications and venous thrombosis.

Miss Cash is working in full co-operation with the surgeons at a hospital where all these growing points of surgery are represented and practised, and where, every day, much new knowledge is being gained. It is right and proper, then, that she should record in book form the points of her wide experience and new ideas. Her former book *A Textbook of Medical Conditions for Physiotherapists* dealt mainly with medical ward problems: the present volume is particularly for use in connection with surgical treatment. It is authoritative and right up-to-date, and contains sections on the breast, lungs, heart, abdomen, peripheral vascular disease, kidneys, etc. It will, therefore, fill a much wanted need, and should be as popular as her other book.

F. A. R. STAMMERS

5

Preface to First Edition

The object of this book is to try to show why physiotherapy is of value in some of the diseases and injuries treated by the surgeon. In most surgical conditions, the purpose of physiotherapy is to assist in the prevention or treatment of complications; for this reason it is the complications rather than the diseases which have been discussed. It was felt that with an understanding of these, much of the work which is so often considered routine would become more interesting and would be carried out far more effectively.

The author has not included a section on congenital or acquired deformities or such orthopaedic procedures as arthroplasty and arthrodesis, as she originally intended to do, because it appeared that a separate book would be needed to cover this work and in addition methods are changing so rapidly that much would be out of date before it could be published.

J.E.C.

Preface to Third Edition

When beginning to prepare a third edition of this textbook it became clear that I would not be able to bring it up-to-date satisfactorily since no one person could make a sufficiently full study of the advances which have taken place in recent years in all the different fields of physiotherapy. The sections on general surgery, neurological and thoracic surgery have, therefore, been completely rewritten by physiotherapists who have specialized in these fields. Mr Brian Day, FRCS, kindly undertook the supervision of the material for the new edition and also added new matter himself especially in the chapters on recent injuries. Mrs Sylvia Cunningham originally proposed the names of the various contributors and initiated the contributors' work.

I would like to express my grateful thanks to Mr Day and to the other contributors, Miss Hamilton, Miss Newton, Miss Shotton, Miss Sutcliffe and Miss Symons, for all the care and interest they have taken. Particularly, I wish to thank Miss P. Jean Cunningham. She had the difficult task of collaborating with people willing to rewrite the various sections and then reconciling the different points of view of the original author and the new contributors. I am very grateful to her. Without her hard work this third edition could never have been produced.

December 1965   J.E.C.

Preface to Fifth Edition

This edition has been completely revised and many changes have been made. Chapters on Thoracic and Cardiac surgery have been omitted since these have been dealt with in a separate book. For the same reason there has been some alteration in the Neurosurgery section. Gynaecological conditions have been dealt with in greater detail as it was felt that there was a need for more information on these subjects, since in the Gynaecological and Obstetric departments in some hospitals physiotherapy is being used more fully. The Recent Injury section has been completely rewritten and it is hoped that the new form will prove more helpful for students of physiotherapy.

The editor would like to give a very sincere welcome to the new contributors. She feels she owes a deep debt of gratitude to all the authors. They have been so generous both in their time and in their co-operation and interest and she would like to take this opportunity to express her very real thanks.

Miss Cash also wishes to thank Mrs Audrey Besterman for the illustrations which have been done with so much care and interest, and Miss P. Jean Cunningham and Miss Heather Potter of Faber & Faber Ltd who have worked hard on the manuscript and have shown unvarying patience and kindness.

Miss Cash would also like to thank Miss D. Caney and Miss M. K. Patrick and all her friends, ex-colleagues and students, too numerous to mention, without whose support and help this book would never have been written or revised. The book is as much theirs and the contributors' as it is hers.

July 1975   J.E.C.

9

Acknowledgements

Mrs M. C. Balfour, who wrote Chapters 4 and 5 on Surgical Neurology, would like to thank Professor Gillingham, Mr Harris and all other Members of the Staff of the Surgical Neurology Department of the Western General Hospital, Edinburgh, for their invaluable help and encouragement.

Mrs Barkway and Miss Coles wish to express their thanks to all those who have helped them in the revision of Chapters 1 and 2. Especially they would like to thank Dr Peter Baskett, Consultant Anaesthetist, Mr Andrew Fox, and Dr H. Eckert, Consultant in Radiotherapy, of the United Bristol Hospitals.

Miss Buston and Miss Cash would like to thank Mr P. Bicknell, Consultant Ear, Nose and Throat Surgeon, the United Bristol Hospitals, for his help and interest in the revision of Chapter 6.

Miss Cash would also wish to express her thanks to Miss Catrin Williams, Consultant Ear, Nose and Throat Surgeon, and Miss Vera Jones, Senior Physiotherapist, H. M. Stanley Hospital, St Asaph, for giving up their time to advise and answer questions.

Miss B. Davis wishes to thank Mr Vitali, FRCS, Principal Medical Officer, Limb Fitting Centre, Roehampton; Miss M. Lynch, MCSP, Superintendent Physiotherapist, Queen Mary's Hospital, Roehampton; Miss M. D. Gardiner, FCSP; and Miss M. A. Mendez, MAOT, Group Head Occupational Therapist to the Westminster Hospital Group, for reading the manuscript and giving much helpful advice. Thanks are also due to Mr N. Bailey, photographic department of the Limb Fitting Centre, Roehampton, for his assistance, and not least, to all patients who so readily agreed to be photographed. Finally, thanks to Mrs M.

Acknowledgements

Lay, who so cheerfully undertook typing Chapter 12.

Mrs Harrison would like to express her gratitude to Mr J. A. Carron Brown, Consultant Obstetrician and Gynaecologist to the United Norwich Hospitals, who has helped her at every stage in the production of Chapter 3, giving of his time most generously; also to Mr R. Burn of the Medical Illustration Unit of the Norfolk and Norwich Hospital for the photographs. Other colleagues have assisted her by their suggestions and advice and in this connection she is indebted to Mr A. Byles, Consultant Obstetrician and Gynaecologist, Mrs R. Gill, Physiotherapist, Mrs D. Suckling, Medical Social Worker, Miss L. Dennes, Ward Sister, and the Reverend P. Morgan, Chaplain. Finally to the editor for her encouragement.

Miss Patrick would like to thank the Medical Staff of the Accident and Surgery Department of the General Hospital, Birmingham, for their help and encouragement in the preparation of the Recent Injury section of this book. She wishes also to express her gratitude to Miss D. Caney, Principal, School of Physiotherapy, Queen Elizabeth Hospital, and her Staff and to all the physiotherapists of the United Birmingham Hospitals, for their help and interest.

Contents

Contents

Plates

15

Figures

Figures

Contributors

Mrs M. C. Balfour, MCSP
formerly Senior Physiotherapist
Department of Surgical Neurology
Western General Hospital, Edinburgh

Mrs B. R. Barkway, MCSP
Deputy Superintendent Physiotherapist
Bristol Royal Infirmary

Miss W. M. Buston, MCSP
Superintendent Physiotherapist
Royal United Hospital, Bath

Miss R. M. Coles, MCSP
Superintendent Physiotherapist
Bristol Royal Infirmary

Miss B. C. Davis, MCSP
Superintendent Physiotherapist
D.H.S.S. Limb Fitting Centre
Queen Mary's Hospital, Roehampton

Mrs S. M. Harrison, MCSP
Senior Obstetric Physiotherapist
Norfolk and Norwich Hospital, Norwich

Miss M. K. Patrick, OBE, MCSP
Superintendent Physiotherapist
The General Hospital, Birmingham

19

CHAPTER 1

Complications Common to all Operations

revised by R. M. COLES, MCSP

No matter how simple and straightforward an operation, or how physically fit the patient when he undergoes it, there are always certain risks which cannot be avoided, though preventive measures can lessen their possibility. These complications which may follow surgery are given here in their order of importance to the physiotherapy student. This is not necessarily the order in which they endanger life.

Respiratory problems

Whenever a general anaesthetic has to be used and morphia is administered, there is the possibility of respiratory problems because these depress the cough reflex. Thoracic surgery and high abdominal surgery are most likely to give rise to chest complications.

Thrombosis

Thrombosis, which may lead to fatal pulmonary or cerebral embolism, is always a postoperative danger. The physiotherapist may easily be the person who discovers this during an exercise period, so must always be watchful for the symptoms.

Wound infections

These are very common due to the prevalence of resistant bacteria. Infections occur even in clean, cold surgery and despite the existence in most large hospitals of teams whose task it is to combat infection.

Pressure sores

Any patient confined to bed must be watched constantly by all who care for him to prevent pressure sores occurring. These may have been precipitated by pressure whilst on the operating table or they may occur later. Pressure can also be caused from within the tissues, i.e. by the presence of oedema. Vigilance is especially needed where the patient is old, unconscious, immobile or incontinent.

Haemorrhage

Another complication is haemorrhage. This can be primary, occurring within the first 24 hours, or secondary, when it can take place up to three weeks postoperatively.

Muscle wasting and impairment of function

If incisions are very extensive and divide, or in extreme cases damage, muscle or nerve tissue, there can be resultant muscle wasting and impairment of function. This can lead to faulty posture, deformities and, rarely, stiff joints.

Cardiac arrest

The ultimate complication is cardiac arrest, and unless immediate action is taken, the symptoms are irreversible. It is therefore vital that it should be recognized at once by everyone who comes in contact with the patient, and that the appropriate action is known and instantly followed.

RESPIRATORY PROBLEMS

Respiratory complications are liable to follow any operation in which general anaesthetics are used. They are clearly likely to be most common in thoracic surgery since in most cases the lungs are already involved. After thoracic surgery the highest incidence is probably in abdominal operations, particularly those which require a supra-umbilical incision.

The two main complications are *bronchitis* and *postoperative lung collapse*. These may lead to bronchopneumonia, bronchiectasis or lung abscess. The factors which predispose towards these complications are increased formation of secretions and decreased ability to eliminate them. The increased secretions may be due to slight irritation of the bronchial mucous membrane by the anaesthetic. Sometimes the mucus formed is stringy and viscid in type and consequently particularly difficult to eliminate. In addition, it is possible that septic material may be inhaled from the nose or throat. This may set up inflammation and further secretion. Very occasionally, if a tube is not passed through the oesophagus prior to operations on the intestine, pressure on the stomach may cause gastric secretions to travel along the oesophagus and these may be inhaled into the lungs while, if the patient is not very carefully watched, postoperative vomiting may result in inhalation of vomitus.

Normally secretions are eliminated by means of the action of the cilia lining the mucous membrane and by the cough reflex. The cilia are, however, inhibited in their movement by the anaesthetic and the cough reflex is depressed by postoperative analgesics. If, in addition, the operation is thoracic or abdominal, coughing is voluntarily inhibited through fear of pain. Coughing is difficult in supine lying, but is perfectly possible in the crook side-lying position and this is a necessary position in order to drain the lungs.

If secretions collect they may form a plug which can block one of the bronchi or bronchioles, obstructing air entry or exit from the lobules distal to the obstruction. Air is then gradually absorbed from the alveoli of these lobules and the area collapses. One of two events may then occur: the mucus plug may become infected and inflammation may spread to the walls of the tubes, setting up a bronchopneumonia, or the bronchioles just proximal to the block may dilate and a bronchiectasis result.

The drop in vital capacity, which inevitably follows operations on the thorax or abdomen, is a further factor in predisposing towards these complications. The diaphragm is responsible for as much as 60% of the normal respiratory movements, but, in the first 24 hours after the operation, its movement may be only 20% of the normal. The result of this fact is that the lungs, particularly the bases, are not fully ventilated and the circulation is slowed, with consequent congestion. Not only is the vitality of the lung lowered, but there may be increased filtration of tissue fluid and slight oedema of the lung bases.

Collapse of part of a lung usually occurs within 24 to 48 hours of the operation and will be suspected if there is a sudden rise of temperature, pulse and respiratory rates, dyspnoea, sometimes cyanosis and diminished movement of the chest wall. Pneumonia occurs after a rather longer interval, usually three or four days. The temperature rise is more gradual, but eventually high, and there is a productive cough.

Physiotherapy

Treatment for chest complications is mainly preventive, though naturally, if complications have arisen, attention will be directed towards their cure. Clearly, if the main cause of chest complications is lowered vital capacity and accumulation of secretions through decreased cough and diminished respiratory movements, the purpose of physiotherapy is to raise vital capacity, stimulate coughing and encourage full use of the lungs. In cases where elimination of mucus is difficult, it is a further object to assist in its removal so that bronchoscopy will not be necessary.

Since vital capacity is lowered, the first principle of treatment is *to train the patient to use the lungs, especially the lower areas, fully.*
TEACHING THE PATIENT TO BREATHE
This is not easy if the patient is still hazy from the anaesthetic and in some discomfort. It is important, therefore, to train good breathing *before* the operation. Particular stress is laid on gaining good inspiration and on the ability to perform diaphragmatic and lower lateral costal breathing at will. An understanding of the value of the correct breathing is essential, so that the patient will co-operate as soon as he recovers from the anaesthetic.

The second principle of treatment is based on the likelihood of secretions accumulating.
COUGHING
The patient must be taught how to cough with as little strain and pain as possible. He must also be taught deep breathing so that the movement of air will help to drive out mucus. These again are best taught pre-operatively. Two points require stress in teaching coughing. Firstly, strain on the wound will be relieved if the patient supports the operation site with his hands and if the knees are drawn up and trunk bent slightly towards the area of the incision (see Plate 3/1). Secondly,

following an inspiration, a short sharp expiration produces the easiest and most effective cough.

In order to facilitate the removal of mucus the secretions of the lungs must be kept moist. *Humidification* can be achieved in several ways:

(*i*) The simplest method is by Tinct. Benzoin. Co. (friar's balsam) inhalations given three times a day. Preferably it should be done immediately before chest physiotherapy is carried out.

(*ii*) Humidifiers which add water, usually warmed, to the oxygen or air which the patient breathes.

(*iii*) In the case of tracheostomy, saline may be injected into the trachea.

(*iv*) By the use of a Wright's nebulizer. In this method a bronchodilator, e.g. salbutamol (Ventolin), or a mucolytic agent can be nebulized for inhalation. Indications for use are bronchospasm or to thin down mucoid sputum.

When, in spite of adequate coughing and practice of breathing exercises, mucus does collect and there is danger of collapse then a third principle applies:

MECHANICAL ASSISTANCE OF ELIMINATION OF MUCUS

This is carried out by means of percussion, resisted breathing, vibrations and postural drainage. There is usually no reason why a patient should not be posturally drained to clear the basal segments of the lungs. However, in certain conditions, such as hypertension, hiatus hernia and some aortic surgery it is contra-indicated. For this reason the physiotherapist must make quite sure of the condition from which the patient is suffering and that the patient she is treating postoperatively is not hypertensive.

If the patient is being nursed in the half-lying position, back rest and pillows may be removed and the crook lying and crook side-lying positions may be taken up, while the foot of the bed can be raised on the bed elevator. Breathing exercises and percussion will be given in these positions. Incidentally, movement and percussion usually help to relieve the flatulence which so often causes abdominal distension and further hampers breathing.

One of the most important points to bear in mind is that the practice of breathing exercises once daily is useless. If they are to be effective in preventing chest complications, they must be used all day long until good breathing becomes a habit. Much depends, therefore, on the ability of the physiotherapist to gain the patient's interest, understanding and co-operation. Frequent short visits are essential, until it is clear that the patient is sufficiently enthusiastic to work on his own.

In circumstances where the patient is unable to cough up the mucus with the aid of physiotherapy for any reason, e.g. inability to co-operate, or weakness such that he cannot cough, laryngoscopy may be performed to suck out the collected secretions. This is often done in conjunction with chest physiotherapy. Very occasionally bronchoscopy may be required. If repeated laryngoscopy or bronchoscopy are needed, it is more likely that an endotracheal tube will be introduced, or tracheostomy performed. By either means the secretions can be removed with suction.

If major chest problems are anticipated pre-operatively, a primary tracheostomy may be performed, e.g. in some cases of cardiac surgery. In other cases it may be necessary to perform tracheostomy post-operatively if the patient's condition does not allow him to co-operate actively in the clearance of copious or viscid secretions.

Chest physiotherapy is continued, the patient being postured to drain the affected segments of the lung or lungs. Percussion, vibrations and rib-springing are used. The patient is asked to attempt to cough, if he is conscious, then the secretions are removed by suction through the tracheostomy. This is carried out as a sterile technique.

The patient who has a tracheostomy needs to be treated regularly at least three or four times per day while the lung is collapsed or the secretions thick and infected. Besides suction given at these times by the physiotherapist, the nursing staff will be sucking out the secretions at, for example, quarter-hourly intervals.

THROMBOSIS AND EMBOLISM

Thrombosis may occur following any operation, though it is probably most common after operations on the pelvis. It tends to occur at any time between the first and twenty-first postoperative day. It is important to realize that there are two distinct types of thrombosis. In one type the vein, often the long saphenous, becomes inflamed and consequently the blood within it rapidly clots. This type is known as a *thrombophlebitis*. In the second variety thrombosis precedes inflammation. This is known as a *phlebothrombosis*. Of the two types the second is by far the more serious because it arises silently, causing no symptoms, and the first evidence that it has occurred may be a pulmonary or cerebral embolism.

Thrombophlebitis

The probable cause of this is damage to the vein wall. In operative surgery the most likely cause is the insertion of an intravenous drip. The vein is irritated and becomes inflamed and the blood rapidly clots. The clot becomes adherent to the vein wall and, since the vein is temporarily obliterated by the clot, embolism, though possible, is unlikely. In many cases the inflammation spreads to the surrounding tissues, and a cellulitis is evident. As the vein is nearly always a superficial one, there will be redness in the region of the vein, and the area will be painful and exquisitely tender to touch and may show considerable oedema. Usually the patient's temperature will rise, largely as a result of the absorption of toxic products produced by the disintegration of the clotted blood.

The inflammatory condition gradually resolves if the irritant is removed, and in many cases the clot is absorbed by the action of phagocytic cells. The vein becomes once more patent. Sometimes, however, organization of the clotted blood takes place by growth into it from the vessel wall of fibroblasts and capillary loops, and the vein becomes changed into a fibrous cord. This is of little significance, since there is a very extensive venous collateral circulation and adequate venous drainage will be established by other veins.

It will be realized that the presence of thrombophlebitis is not dangerous to life though it may be very uncomfortable for the patient. Treatment is, therefore, directed to aiding resolution of the cellulitis and to relieving discomfort. If the cause is an intravenous drip, it will for obvious reasons be removed and only inserted elsewhere if necessary.

PHYSIOTHERAPY
Physiotherapy can help to fulfil the objects of treatment mainly by the application of heat to the area of cellulitis. Both shortwave diathermy and inductothermy prove most effective; inflammation rapidly subsides and pain and tenderness disappear. Usually no other treatment is necessary. If movements were being given at the time of onset they should be continued.

Phlebothrombosis

This type of thrombosis tends to start in the veins of the foot and calf, sometimes spreading to the larger popliteal, femoral and iliac veins. The cause is still not fully understood, but there are a number of possible explanations.

(*i*) *Following surgery there is a rise in the number of platelets and amount of fibrinogen in the blood.* The greater the handling of the tissues and the longer the operation the greater will be the platelet and fibrinogen content and the more likelihood of thrombosis.

(*ii*) A second very important factor is the *altered speed of blood flow.* If the flow is slow there is a tendency for platelets to fall out of the stream and in addition thromboplastic substances are not so readily carried away. Following surgery flow tends to be slowed. Postoperative sedation, abdominal distension, faulty posture with hips and knees bent, diminished muscle contractions, reduced respiratory excursion will all affect the venous return.

(*iii*) A third factor is *minor intimal damage.* This may happen during the operation and until the patient recovers consciousness and begins to move about. The deep muscle relaxation, if the legs are resting flat on the table or bed, causes excessive pressure on the veins producing ischaemia and damage to the vein walls.

When these factors are present, platelets adhere to the site of the damage. There is a release of thromboplastic substances and fibrin is formed. Red and white cells are caught up in the fibrin network.

The speed at which the thrombus builds up depends on the rate of blood flow. If the flow is slow the thromboplastic substances are not carried away and more fibrin is formed, the thrombus developing quickly and sometimes extending for a considerable distance along the vein as a 'tail' floating freely within the vein. Gradually the thrombus becomes canalized by the growth into it of endothelial cells. It is also organized by the penetration of cells from the deeper part of the vein wall. The latter process is speeded up by the fact that the presence of the developing thrombus irritates and sets up inflammation of the wall. Occasionally this inflammation spreads to the surrounding tissue involving the adjacent artery and causing arterial spasm.

Early diagnosis of the condition is vital because of the danger of break-off of the thrombus before it becomes adherent, or of the 'tail', leading to embolism. The earliest signs are tenderness on palpation of the calf, a slight rise in temperature and pulse rate and sometimes pain in the calf muscles on dorsiflexion of the foot with the knee straight. After a few days signs of venous obstruction may appear. Oedema develops in the foot round the ankle, masking the extensor tendons and filling out the hollows, and the superficial veins appear fuller. If the vein is inflamed there may be pain and cramp in the calf and tenderness over the vein.

If the thrombosis extends into the femoral or iliac veins the whole leg becomes oedematous and sometimes it is pale and cold, possibly the result of arterial spasm.

TREATMENT

Attempts are made to avoid thrombosis by protection of the deep veins during the period of surgery and unconsciousness. The ankles are supported on sandbags so that pressure is taken off the calves and the legs are elevated until the patient is moving actively.

A careful watch is kept for early signs and the physiotherapist is expected to check for tenderness in the calf and discomfort on dorsiflexion of the foot. As soon as the onset of thrombosis is detected anticoagulants are given and usually physiotherapy is continued; however, it must be ascertained that this is the wish of the surgeon in charge of the case.

The usual immediate treatment is by heparin drip; this is necessary as oral anticoagulants are not effective for 48 hours. The clotting time will be carefully monitored for several days, often up to seven. The drip may be continued for five to seven days and often the patient is ambulant during this time, taking his drip stand with him as he walks. The time in bed is always as short as possible, often only one to two days. While in bed breathing and leg exercises will be continued. When he is allowed up the patient must wear an elastic bandage on the affected leg. This begins at the toes, must include the heel and must be firmly and frequently reapplied.

If the thrombosis extends to the femoral vein, swelling is unlikely ever to subside completely. Physiotherapy is then given with the object of reducing oedema, preventing organization, and strengthening the leg muscle pump. It will follow the lines indicated for a gravitational ulcer (for details see Chapter 20 of *A Textbook of Medical Conditions for Physiotherapists*, fifth edition).

Embolism

Embolism may be another serious complication, the two sites being the pulmonary and the cerebral vessels. *Pulmonary embolism* most commonly follows a phlebothrombosis. Part of the thrombus may become detached from the vein wall or part of the 'tail' may break off. The embolus then passes in the bloodstream, through the heart, into the pulmonary circulation.

Embolism may be due to one large embolus or multiple small emboli. If large, the thrombus may 'stick' at the bifurcation of the pulmonary artery, roll up into a ball and completely obstruct all blood entry into the lungs. The patient will then die within seconds. If rather smaller, the clot may block one of the two vessels and one lung will fail to receive blood. If the patient is young and fit, he may survive with one lung out of action. The embolus may of course be much smaller, or there may be multiple small emboli, blocking only small branches, and the patient who is suddenly stricken with pain in the chest and spitting of blood will recover, but will be left with a small infarct which will gradually be converted into scar tissue.

Cerebral embolism appears to be particularly liable to occur after a mitral valvotomy, or oesophagectomy or pneumonectomy. The signs and symptoms vary with the size of the vessel blocked and the site of the embolism. There may therefore be a transient loss of consciousness with rapid and full recovery, or, on the other hand, the patient, if he survives, may be left with a hemiplegia.

PHYSIOTHERAPY

A severe pulmonary embolism is likely to prove fatal, but in the case of small or multiple emboli when physiotherapy is already being given for the particular operation, physiotherapy will continue, but if the patient is getting up he will probably now be confined to bed for one to three days. It is most important, however, that the circulation should be stimulated and the legs exercised, and full activity in bed, together with breathing exercises should be stressed.

More treatment is needed if the patient recovers from a cerebral embolism but is left with disabilities such as a hemiplegia. Physiotherapy is then required for the weakness or loss of voluntary movement. This treatment will be conducted on the usual lines for the condition except that progress may be delayed as a result of the original condition. If, for example, the cerebral embolism has followed a mitral valvotomy, the patient may not be allowed to get up to start the usual walking re-education at the third or fourth day, but may be confined to bed for longer. Passive movements can however be started at once and a start may be made on active re-education. When the patient is allowed to get up and walk, the routine training in balance, getting up from a chair and sitting down, and walking as used for hemiplegia, will be begun.

UNHEALED WOUNDS AND INFECTION

Surgical incisions will heal quickly and with little formation of scar tissue under suitable conditions. There must be adequate apposition of the tissues and an adequate supply of blood containing the substances necessary for repair. Excessive strain on the site of incision, such as might result from constant coughing, must not occur, though healing is stimulated by some pull on the wound, provided that it is not excessive. It is safe to say that a wound will not break down, unless it is inadequately sutured or unless it becomes infected.

Infection is sadly not at all rare and cannot be eliminated from operating theatres. Resistant strains of bacteria are becoming much more common, especially in hospitals, and an already unwell patient who contracts an infection from, for example, *Staphylococcus aureus*, which may be only sensitive to one or two antibiotics, can be in a critical condition. Most hospitals have a special team working exclusively on the control of infection and their advice is readily available and should be sought in all cases of wound infection.

The presence of infection in a previously clean wound may be recognized by the fact that the wound becomes painful, throbs and is very tender. The temperature of the area rises and sometimes redness and oedema may be seen around the wound; the sutures then tend to cut through the tissues and the wound to gape either in its whole length or between the sutures.

Healing is likely to be less satisfactory if the area is already infected. The presence of sepsis necessitating operation, as for example in the case of a gangrenous appendix, or in empyema, involves the use of drainage tubes to permit free drainage of the pus and ensure healing from the base upwards. If tubes remain in for any length of time they are apt to cause irritation of the walls of the track with consequent fibrous tissue formation; then healing becomes difficult when the tube is eventually removed. In addition where tissues are damaged and there is sepsis, the proteolytic ferments, liberated by bacteria and phagocytic cells, tend to digest the tissues in the region of the wound and may do so for a considerable distance. This loss of tissue must be replaced by granulations which will later become converted into scar tissue. For these reasons, tubes are usually shortened quickly and removed as soon as possible, usually between three and seven days.

In the case of incisions of the abdominal wall, abdominal distension might cause bursting either of the whole wound or areas between the sutures. Persistent distension is therefore to be avoided.

If, as a result of these factors, scarring occurs in the musculature of, say, the walls of the abdominal or pelvic cavities, then there is always the possibility of protrusion of the contents of the cavity through the weakened area. This condition is known as *incisional hernia*.

It will be seen from these facts that certain points are very important when dealing with wounds of operative surgery. The most important point is obviously to obtain quick healing without infection. To obtain this, great care is necessary in dressing the wound. If a wound becomes infected, steps should be taken to allow free drainage and stimulate healing.

PHYSIOTHERAPY
Firstly, active exercises are good, since, as has already been seen, some strain on the wound stimulates the healing process. Excessive strain is of course to be avoided; therefore an abdominal operation should not be followed by outer range abdominal exercises or heavy work such as double hip and knee flexion.

Secondly, if a clean wound becomes infected, cleaning may be assisted and subsequent healing stimulated by the use of some form of dry heat. If the infection is superficial, infra-red or radiant heat are satisfactory, but if the infection is deep-seated, shortwave therapy should be used. In the first case, treatment is usually only given after the sutures have been cut and the wound allowed to gape so that free drainage is established. In either case treatment should be given at least twice daily.

Since the healing of wounds which are either slow to heal or which required resuturing is characterized by the formation of much scar tissue, certain after-effects may be noticed. Firstly, the scar may be an unsightly keloid one, in which the scar is red, raised and puckered.

This is a contra-indication to physiotherapy, as massage and active exercises are usually found to stimulate the production of more scar tissue.

Secondly, the scar will be adherent to underlying tissue and will probably hamper movement. It may also cause discomfort, as it pulls on other tissues. Not only will it be adherent, but it may well contract and produce deformity. Therefore, as soon as the wound is firmly healed, massage with lanolin should be used. It should be carried out over the surface of the scar to try to loosen it from the underlying tissue.

For particularly hard scars, such as sometimes occur after release of the flexor retinaculum in the carpal tunnel syndrome or after operation for Dupuytren's contracture, ultrasound therapy is helpful. On suitable areas, paraffin wax treatment nearly always results in scars becoming softer and more elastic. The sooner the treatment can be started, the more successful it will be.

Occasionally a scar may be painful, probably because a superficial nerve has become caught up in the fibrous tissue. Different measures have been advocated for this complication. One principle is to soften the fibrous tissue. Pain may then be relieved. This is often successfully done by X-ray irradiation. Alternatively, the fibrous tissue may be excised and the nerve freed. Physiotherapy then has no place in the treatment.

PRESSURE SORES

Pressure sores can be divided into superficial and deep sores. Superficial sores begin in the skin. These break down leaving a shallow, painful ulcer. Deep sores begin in the subcutaneous tissues. Muscle and fat have less resistance to pressure than skin, and destruction may occur in these while the skin covering them shows only erythema. Eventually the skin breaks down and the deeper necrosed tissues are exposed. Both types of sore are due to pressure. This drives the blood out of the vessels and deprives the tissue of nutrition. In a patient with normal sensation the pressure causes discomfort and he alters his position to relieve this, but if there is loss of sensation or he is unconscious or too ill to move pressure will not be relieved.

Other factors which may precipitate sores are: (i) ill-fitting splints; (ii) friction from rucked sheets; (iii) persistent soaking of the skin resulting from incontinence and also from poor skin.

Likely sites for pressure sores are the heels, malleoli, great tro-chanters, elbows and sacrum. In the latter case, if a patient is nursed in a propped up position he tends to slide down and this causes a shearing force on the sacral area, rupturing deeper tissues and small blood vessels and consequently leading to a deep pressure sore.

Treatment

Pressure sores should not be allowed to develop. They can usually be prevented by ensuring that unconscious patients or those suffering from loss of sensation do not suffer from prolonged pressure. If the patient is confined to bed and unable to help himself, he must be turned every two to three hours night and day. If he is up, sitting in a chair, he has to be taught to relieve pressure by lifting himself up by his arms, at first every ten minutes and later at regular intervals. Care is also taken to see that splints do not rub, sheets are smooth, the patient does not slide down in bed and the skin is kept dry. The skin is washed with warm water and rubbed with a good barrier cream.

Sheepskins are frequently used under the helpless or heavy patient to prevent friction and therefore to eliminate one cause of chafing and soreness of the skin. The lanolin content of the sheepskin is also beneficial to the possibly poor skin.

Ripple beds, in which the areas of pressure on the patient's body are constantly changed, are another aid to prevention of sores, but do not supersede good nursing and regular turning.

Once a sore has developed, all pressure must be taken off it until it has healed. This will involve the use of special packs and mattresses. The actual sore is treated by excision of any slough, antibiotics in solution to clear up infection and wet sterile saline dressings, covered with a dry dressing and sealed off with a porous Elastoplast.

PHYSIOTHERAPY

This can help in the prevention and in the treatment of sores. When treating any patient liable to develop pressure sores the physiothera-pist should examine the skin carefully, and immediately any redness appears, the heels, sacrum or whatever area is involved should be rubbed with an ice-cube. This must be done at least twice daily.

If a sore has developed, a course of ultraviolet and infra-red rays will help to control infection and stimulate healing.

Should a sore become infected it is most probable that there will be a slough adherent to the floor of the sore, and this can be removed by obtaining a very severe reaction with ultraviolet rays. A strong dose is essential for this purpose and should be obtained with the Kromayer lamp, placed so close to the sore that it is just not touching it. In this way, no rays will be absorbed in the air, and all of them will be used to obtain the desired circulatory reaction. If the sore is large it is possible to irradiate the whole area at once by using the Alpine Sun lamp at a distance of 12 or 18 inches (30 or 46 cm). In addition, the shorter abiotic rays will be absorbed in the slough itself and will destroy a certain number of bacteria, but unless the slough is very thin, the effect on the bacteria as a whole is likely to be negligible. As the slough absorbs so many rays, few will actually reach the tissues beneath, and it is necessary to give a much stronger dose than usual in order to produce sufficient reaction in the tissues lying beneath.

It is not possible to treat any of the surrounding skin as this strong dose would produce a blister; therefore, it is necessary for the skin to be screened right up to the edges of the wound with sterile Vaseline petroleum jelly and gauze.

If the slough is very thick, or consists of hardened gangrenous tissue, no ultraviolet rays will be able to penetrate to the bed, but a dose to the surrounding skin may produce sufficient vascular changes beneath the slough to be effective. A second or third degree dose should be given.

The effect of this treatment is to increase the blood supply and the ability to fight the infection. It is also of value in that it will produce sufficient exudate to cause increased pressure from within and so force the slough away from its bed. This will free it, so that it can eventually be removed. If treatment has been effective, the dressing will be coated with thickened, yellowish pus and the floor of the sore will look pink and clean.

HAEMORRHAGE

Haemorrhage may complicate any operation, but it is particularly liable to occur when surgery has been necessary in a very vascular area, such as the thyroid gland or tonsils. If bleeding is excessive or prolonged, various signs and symptoms will arise. The pulse will be feeble, the blood pressure low, and respirations fast and often of the sighing type. The skin will become cold and clammy and the complexion and mucous membranes pale. The patient will be restless, feel thirsty and complain of faintness and giddiness.

Should haemorrhage occur, physical treatment is immediately stopped and first-aid treatment given until further help can be obtained. If possible the patient should be placed in the lying position and if the bleeding is external, digital pressure may be applied above the site of haemorrhage. The main measures are, however, precautionary. If there is any reason to suspect the possibility of haemorrhage, as for example, where there is sepsis, vigorous movements between the third and fourteenth days should be avoided.

MUSCLE ATROPHY AND IMBALANCE

Muscles may be in poor condition, as regards both tone and bulk, before an operation is undertaken, or they may be in excellent condition, but affected by the operation. Into the first group comes the elderly patient whose muscles are weak and flabby, and the patient who has been ill for some time, possibly suffering from nutritional disturbances such as might be present in gastric or duodenal ulcer. Again there is the bronchiectatic child or adult whose musculature is poor.

In the second group, muscles may be affected both generally and locally by surgery. Most operations demand a certain amount of lessening of general activity. This is as true for the meniscectomy as for the serious pelvic or brain operation. This inactivity is often increased by fear. The effect of muscular activity on the blood vessels is diminished, venous return is lessened, cardiac output is correspondingly reduced and the normally freely circulating oxygenated blood is available in smaller quantities for all the muscles; consequently their metabolism is reduced and their bulk and power diminished.

For several reasons muscles in the region of the operation may very easily be affected. Sometimes muscles are deliberately cut, though often this is avoided. No real harm results from this if they are adequately sutured, though a small amount of scar tissue must result. This, however, will not markedly reduce the power if it is kept supple. On the other hand some exudate and haemorrhage may occur, and if this is likely to be considerable, Redivac drains are inserted and maintained for 24 to 48 hours, so that the haematoma is drained away and the tissues remain soft.

The nerve supply to the muscles may be damaged at the time of operation, though this is always avoided where possible. For example, in surgery of the cervical lymph glands, the accessory nerve is occasionally damaged and trapezius and sternomastoid may both be affected. Again, in a thyroidectomy, it is difficult to avoid the recurrent laryngeal nerve and the muscles of the larynx may then be weakened. In cholecystectomy the ninth, tenth and eleventh intercostal nerves may all be severed and marked weakness of one side of the abdominal wall will result.

Occasionally, stretching of, or pressure on one or more nerves may occur. If the relaxant drugs such as curare are used during the operation there is complete absence of tone in the muscles, and consequently no protection for the nerves. If a position is necessary in which pressure on a nerve might occur, there is a greater tendency for a paresis to result. If an Esmarch's rubber bandage around the thigh is used for a tourniquet in operations on the knee, a drop foot occasionally occurs, probably owing to ischaemia of the lateral popliteal nerve. This neurological damage means atrophy of the muscles with diminished or lost tone and reduced or absent power, according to the extent of the lesion.

In some operations certain positions may be necessary which prevent active use of the muscles. In operations for recurrent dislocation of the shoulder, for example, the arm may be fixed in adduction and medial rotation. This lack of movement must inevitably result in diminished metabolic processes and therefore in atrophy.

Pain may result in inhibition of muscle, either deliberately through fear, or as a result of reflex action. In cases of operations on joints, distension or damage of the capsule stimulates its nerve endings and reflex inhibition results. This is often seen in operations on the knee or the shoulder. After operations on the spinal cord, patients are afraid to move, especially if much pain in the back or leg has preceded the operation. The result is atrophy of the spinal muscles.

Whatever the cause, it appears that atrophy and hypotonia of muscle will occur following any surgical procedure. The most outstanding effect of this is alteration in posture usually affecting the body as a whole. For example atrophy and hypotonia of the spinal muscles will lead to a loss of the erect carriage of the trunk. If the gluteal muscles are also affected, increased pelvic tilt will be followed by spinal deformity.

When the patient first gets up and begins to walk about, his general posture is likely to be poor; postural flat feet and round shoulders with poking head may be particularly noticeable. Should weakness of the trunk muscles be unilateral then muscle imbalance is particularly noticeable, and may well lead to gross deformity. This is most clearly seen in thoracic operations or in cases of interference with the nerve supply of abdominal muscles. Scoliosis is a very likely result and one which should have been avoided.

Another noticeable effect of muscle atrophy is diminished power, with possible serious results, since the muscles are the first line of defence of the joints. Inadequate muscles will result in continuous minor traumata to joint structures and a chronic synovitis may develop. This is particularly liable to happen if care is not taken following operations on the knee joint.

If the abdominal muscles are the ones to be affected then their function is impaired and not only will posture be disturbed, but they will no longer adequately protect the abdominal viscera or maintain the intra-abdominal pressure. If intra-abdominal pressure drops, then respiration, venous return, defaecation, and support of the abdominal viscera will all be affected. Again, scarring in abdominal muscles means a weak point and may lead to incisional hernia.

Muscle weakness may be one of the factors leading to stiffness of joints. If the muscle has insufficient power to move the joint through its full range, then full range is never attained and adaptive contractures will result.

PHYSIOTHERAPY

Muscle atrophy can usually be avoided except in the case of nerve involvement. The principle is the practice of active contraction, and if possible active exercises, before the operation, immediately after the operation, and for a considerable period after this. All muscle groups should be exercised as vigorously, as often, and in as wide a range as possible. If active movement is impossible then static contractions should be used. For example, in the case of skeletal traction for a fractured tibia or calcaneus, static contractions for all groups, even though the leg cannot be moved, are essential. Where static contractions cannot be obtained, passive exercise, by the use of the faradic current, may be substituted, but it should only be used until active work can be undertaken.

Another important point to be observed is the wearing of shoes, not slippers, to aid good firm gait and correct posture once the patient is ambulant. The feet are frequently painful after bed-rest or varicose vein surgery.

CARDIAC ARREST

Unless immediate action is taken once the diagnosis is made, death is the inevitable result. The main symptoms of this condition are: (*i*) change of colour to blue or white; (*ii*) no pulses felt in radial, femoral or carotid arteries; (*iii*) the patient is unconscious; (*iv*) sometimes the pupils are dilated and fixed. When all these symptoms are present there is no doubt as to the diagnosis.

Treatment should be begun at once and help must be called for. The patient must be placed flat on a firm surface, e.g. a board under the mattress, with the head extended and lower jaw pushed forward. The first operator will begin external cardiac massage. This is done by placing the heels of both hands (with the arms straight), to reinforce one another, over the lower third of the sternum. Very firm pressure is given 50 to 60 times per minute. Periods must be allowed for the lungs to inflate. The second operator will begin artificial ventilation by mouth-to-mouth breathing, preferably with an airway, or if possible with an Air Viva resuscitation bag, in order to give a high concentration of oxygen. This must be done twelve times per minute. The two operations must not be carried out simultaneously and must be in the ratio of five pressures to one blow. The nose should be pinched whilst ventilation is performed.

The board, airway and Air Viva bag are basic resuscitation equipment in most wards.

As soon as the cardiac arrest team arrives, which will probably be within three minutes of calling them, the procedure is:

(*i*) E.C.G. will be set up to determine whether ventricular fibrillation or asystole has been the cause, as treatment depends on this knowledge.

(*ii*) The patient will be intubated.

(*iii*) A drip of bicarbonate of soda to correct the acidosis present will be started.

Ventricular fibrillation will be defibrillated by using an electric defibrillator. Cardiac stimulants will be given for asystole. These may be adrenaline, isoprenaline or calcium chloride.

The patient will be moved to the Intensive Care Unit. Here monitoring of the cardiovascular system and renal output will be instituted.

Respiratory support on a mechanical ventilator may be needed.

A chest X-ray will be taken to ascertain whether there are any fractured ribs with a resultant pneumothorax ensuing from the considerable pressure applied during cardiac massage. Most patients need intravenous mannitol to reduce cerebral oedema.

The physiotherapist will not be required once the resuscitation team arrives, but if she fails to initiate treatment, should the emergency arise, they may be too late to save the patient's life.

TERMS USED TO DESCRIBE CERTAIN SURGICAL PROCEDURES

Certain terms are commonly used to define surgical procedures. In many cases a suffix is attached to the name of the organ or part being treated, and if the suffix is understood, further definition is unnecessary.

The suffix **ectomy** is derived from the Greek word meaning 'a cutting out'. Hence if the colon is removed, we use the word colectomy, or in the case of the stomach, gastrectomy.

The suffix **otomy** is derived from the Greek word meaning 'to cut', and if an incision is made in order to perform a wider operation or to carry out an investigation the suffix may be used. A craniotomy is a cutting into the skull and might be followed by the removal of a cerebral tumour. A thoracotomy is the making of an incision through the chest wall and may be performed for a lobectomy, pneumonectomy or mitral valvotomy.

The suffix **ostomy** is derived from the Greek word meaning 'mouth' and indicates therefore the making of an opening. Colostomy is the formation of an opening through the abdominal wall into the colon, and a suprapubic cystostomy is the forming of an artificial opening through the abdominal wall just above the pubis into the bladder.

The suffix **oscopy** originates from the Greek 'to look' and indicates an inspection of a hollow organ or body cavity by means of an instrument devised for this purpose. The word *endoscopy* is commonly used to describe this process and the instrument is known as the *endoscope*. Often the prefix is altered according to the organ or cavity to be examined in this way. Thus an examination of the more proximal parts of the bronchial tree may be carried out by a bronchoscope and the procedure is known as a bronchoscopy. Similarly the stomach may be examined by gastroscopy, the pleural cavity by thoracoscopy and the bladder by cystoscopy. It is usually possible to withdraw, by suction, material from the walls or lumen of the organ through the endoscope or to insert a knife to scrape the walls or to divide adhesions.

The suffix **ograph(y)** indicates a writing or written description. The process entails, as a rule, the filling of the organ or vessel with a radio-opaque substance, followed by X-ray photographs of the parts. Thus an *angiograph* is a written description of the state of certain vessels seen in the above way; a *cholecystography* is an examination and description of the state of the gall-bladder. The X-ray photograph is usually known as the **'gram'**, hence cystogram, angiogram.

Plasty comes from the Greek word meaning 'to mould' and is usually a suffix indicating that a certain tissue is being repaired, re-modelled or built up. Hence a *pyloroplasty* is a refashioning of the pyloric orifice of the stomach. An *arthroplasty* is the remodelling of a joint, often by means of using other material than body tissue.

The word **resection** is derived from the Latin re = again, and secare = to cut, and indicates the operation of cutting out. Thus a rib resection indicates the removal of a rib, and a resection of the intestine the removal of part of the gut.

Many other words may be used, but these are some of the words most frequently met with.

CHAPTER 2

General Surgery

by B. R. BARKWAY, MCSP, and R. M. COLES, MCSP,

This chapter will deal with the more common surgical procedures which the physiotherapist will encounter in her work on a general surgical ward.

It is the practice in most hospitals for pre- and postoperative physiotherapy to be ordered. The variations of surgery being performed are infinite but all conditions mentioned in this chapter are found routinely and will be treated by the physiotherapist in training.

The physiotherapy which is applicable to all the conditions dealt with in this chapter will be given first; following each surgical procedure any special precautions or points to be stressed will be listed.

PRE-OPERATIVE PHYSIOTHERAPY

The ideal situation would be for every patient undergoing surgery to meet the physiotherapist pre-operatively, and the postoperative regime could then be taught and established, while he felt reasonably fit. This would mean that on the first postoperative day, when he feels at his worst, he does not have to establish a relationship with yet another strange person, however the ideal cannot always happen. Patients are very often not admitted until the evening before surgery, due to pressure on beds, and there are a very large proportion who enter hospital as emergencies. Here of necessity the surgery is performed immediately.

In the case of major general surgery, the patient is usually admitted a few days beforehand. Where this happens the physiotherapist has the opportunity to gain the patient's confidence and to teach him his postoperative routine.

42

Points to be noted pre-operatively

Read the patient's notes. By so doing, not only his immediate need for surgery will be understood, but relevant data, such as previous lung diseases, chronic bronchitis, heart disease or tendency to thrombosis will be learnt. Establish a good rapport with the patient. Discover whether he is a smoker, if so firmly tell him he will help his post-operative recovery if he stops, at least until he is convalescent.

Teach him his postoperative routine. This must include:

EXPLANATION

Give an explanation suited to the patient's intelligence and understanding, of reasons for physiotherapy, i.e. to clear any secretions from the lungs, to maintain full expansion of the lungs, and to maintain good lower limb circulation. Posture and trunk exercises need not be mentioned at this stage.

TO MAINTAIN FULL EXPANSION OF THE LUNGS

Localized breathing is taught, the patient being asked to breathe in against the pressure of the physiotherapist's hands, which give direction and some resistance. Special attention must be given to the lower segments of the lungs. The patient is taught to roll onto each side so that each lung may be treated thoroughly. He is taught to roll in the crook position and to allow his head to flex, so that strain is minimized on the abdominal wall. This is taught as routine since the chest cannot be adequately treated in half-lying or crook-lying.

Coughing. The patient is taught to do this in the crook position and to hold the incision firmly whilst he coughs. The difference between a real cough which can bring up mucus and a mere clearing of the throat which achieves nothing must be stressed. If the patient is known to have any chest problems, e.g. bronchiectasis, he must be given postural drainage, localized breathing, vibrations and percussion for the affected areas at least twice per day.

LEG EXERCISES

These must be kept simple and few in number. In this way the patient is not confused and will remember to perform them. Active foot movements are taught and also quadriceps and gluteal contractions and alternate knee flexion and extension. It must be stressed that the only way for them to be effective is for the patient to practise them frequently, i.e. five minutes every hour. All these can be started on the first postoperative day. It is vital that the patient understands that they will do him no harm, especially knee flexion and extension. He may well have a catheter attached to his leg and will be afraid to move unless he understands that movement will help, not hinder, his recovery.

POSTOPERATIVE PHYSIOTHERAPY

This begins on the first postoperative day, and it will be assumed here that the patient received pre-operative instruction.

Before beginning her treatment the physiotherapist should:

Read the operation notes.

Check blood pressure, pulse rate and temperature.

Ascertain position of drainage tubes, drips, etc.

Check that the patient has received his analgesic cover. The most commonly used drugs are, for example, Omnopon or pethidine. Where drugs are prescribed physiotherapy *should not be given* until the appropriate drugs have been administered, as in major surgery it is far too painful for the patient to co-operate without analgesic cover. *Entonox* is a mixture of nitrous oxide and oxygen. In some hospitals it is administered by physiotherapists and is helpful in the relief of pain after some major surgery.

Postoperatively the *incisions* will be firmly dressed, the dressings held in place by Elastoplast or Netelast, and will always be minimal.

Very frequently the patient will have an intravenous drip of saline/ plasma, a Ryle's tube to remove gastric secretions and a Redivac drain in the incision to minimise haematoma formation. In more severe conditions there may be further drainage tubes, and after some surgery a catheter. It will be realized that in the more minor conditions none of these are required, or at the most only the intravenous drip.

The typical picture presented to the physiotherapist of the patient who has had major surgery will be: the patient is in half-lying with an intravenous drip, Ryle's tube, Redivac drain and possibly a catheter.

It is essential to ask a nurse or colleague to help lower the patient into the lying position. One person supports the patient while the other removes the back rest and all but one pillow. A second pillow is kept in readiness to place behind the patient when he rolls onto his side. As in the pre-operative instruction the patient is asked to flex his head and knees and to allow himself to relax as he rolls.

LOCALIZED RESISTED BREATHING

This is then performed with vibrations on expiration. The basal and posterior segments receive most attention, aiming at the greatest thoracic excursion possible. It is often easier at this stage to get maximum thoracic excursion and maximum air interchange by using lower costal breathing.

After several deep breaths the patient is asked to give a forced expiration; any secretions present can then be heard as well as felt. This may be sufficient to clear secretions which are in the main bronchus and they can be removed without the exertion of coughing. However, a good cough must be achieved to make sure that any mucus present has been removed.

When the physiotherapist is satisfied that one lung is clear of secretions and fully expanding, the patient is helped onto the other side, care being taken that drainage tubes, drips, etc., are not pulled or dragged.

If the leg exercises have been performed first and the patient encouraged to do them frequently himself, it is often a good idea to leave the patient on his side, as he probably finds it a comfortable position as long as he is well supported. Pressure is thus relieved on sacrum, buttocks and heels; and a nursing procedure, visitors, or some other reason will ensure that he is returned to the sitting position by the nursing staff.

It is essential to roll the patient onto *both* sides even though it means lying on the incision. If the incision is, for example, right lateral, it means that during the operation the patient was lying on his left side, therefore this lung is the one in which secretions will have collected, so it is equally as vulnerable to atelectasis as the operated side where respiratory excursion is inhibited by pain due to muscles having been cut.

An experienced physiotherapist can often detect collapse by gentle percussion, or by the patient's inability to hold his breath when asked to do so. Another indication of collapse is if the patient takes a series of small sniffs instead of one firm inspiration when asked to take a deep breath.

Clinically, collapse can be diagnosed by the doctor, or an experienced physiotherapist, who can use a stethoscope, listening to the chest.

X-ray will confirm the clinical diagnosis and show the extent of the collapse.

COUGHING

If during the treatment the secretions have not been cleared through a forced expiration, the patient must then cough. To do this efficiently and with as little pain as possible, the incision must be supported firmly by the patient or physiotherapist and in the case of abdominal surgery the knees must be in the crook position. One good cough following several deep breaths is required. This will remove the mucus effectively without exhausting the patient.

POSTURAL DRAINAGE

This can help to clear the secretions and where collapse has occurred, is essential for the affected area. This is usually perfectly safe, but if in any doubt a check should be made with the houseman or ward sister. Postural drainage is contra-indicated, for example, in hiatus hernia.

LEG EXERCISES

These are given as described in the pre-operative routine. They must be performed frequently to have any useful effect on the circulation; the time in which the circulation is influenced by each session is of only a very short duration, so once or twice a day will not prevent stasis and thrombosis. If the patient complains of calf pain during exercise this must be reported immediately to the Sister or Staff nurse. Single leg movements are best, double leg being too strenuous. Early ambulation quickly replaces leg exercises, the majority of patients being allowed out of bed in 24 or 48 hours.

For the patient who is allowed to sit out but not walk, leg exercises continue to be necessary. Especially he should be encouraged to move his feet vigorously to aid venous return while his legs are in the dependent position.

POSTURE

Patients whilst in bed should be shown how to sit equally on both buttocks and pillows should be firm and even, leaving no gaps into which the lumbar spine can sag.

Once ambulant, patients tend to hug the incision and to flex the spine, so good upright posture must be encouraged.

TRUNK AND ARM EXERCISES

These are necessary in certain conditions. They will be dealt with under the appropriate operations.

WARD CLASSES

These are of very little value except in specific wards where all patients have like conditions, but if there are several patients who all need similar exercises, e.g. arm or posture correction, they can usefully have their physiotherapy together in the day room.

Summary

Wherever possible pre-operative exercises and immediate postoperative treatment should be started. These should include as stated, localized breathing, rolling onto each side, and leg exercises. Early ambulation is encouraged, stitches and clips are removed at seven to ten days. Once out of bed and walking, leg exercises can be discontinued.

Chest physiotherapy is continued just so long as it is necessary, this may be only one to two days, e.g. the young appendicectomy, or it may be until the patient leaves hospital, e.g. the elderly bronchitic. Certainly all patients should be kept on the physiotherapist's list if the temperature remains raised, even though this is possibly due to other causes such as urinary infection or wound infection. Until chest complications are definitely excluded it is safest to check daily.

After minor surgery patients are discharged to convalescence with their stitches in. In all cases they are discharged as soon as possible.

INCISIONS

Figure 2/1 shows some of the common abdominal incisions, the incision for simple mastectomy and for operations on the thyroid gland.

The decision to use any particular incision is a personal one taken by the surgeon. The ideal incision is one which heals satisfactorily, gives direct access to the operation site and minimal inconvenience to the patient.

If, for example, speed is essential in emergency surgery of the stomach and duodenum an *upper midline incision* to just above the umbilicus will be used. There is a minimum of haemorrhage as it is made through the linea alba, the disadvantage being the tendency to heal badly and to result in incisional hernia.

Much more commonly used are *paramedian incisions*, either supra- or sub-umbilical, parallel with the midline and about one inch (2.5 cm) from it, on either right or left. This results in a strong scar. They can

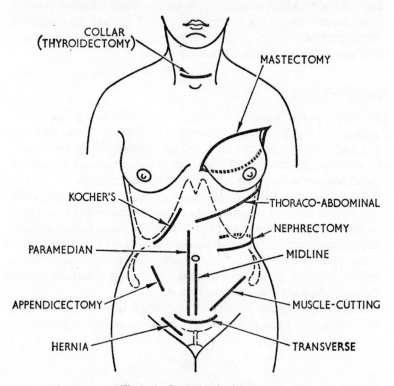

Fig. 2/1 Common incisions.

also be easily extended in contrast with the median (midline) incision which cannot be extended satisfactorily around the umbilicus.

In operations on the thyroid gland the cosmetic result is the top priority so that the *incision chosen will follow the natural creases of the skin of the neck* at approximately one inch (2·5 cm) above the sternum. Similarly in breast surgery the extent and line of the incision chosen now is such that the patient suffers minimal psychological damage from the resulting scar.

It is clear that the best incision will vary from operation to operation and from patient to patient. In the same way there are several different methods of wound closure, each having its own advantages and disadvantages. The skin may be closed with clips, non-absorbable sutures, 'invisible' intradermal absorbable sutures, or with deep sutures passing right through the abdominal wall called 'deep tension' sutures.

From the physiotherapist's point of view it is necessary to know which incision has been used. Although the basic aims and principles of physiotherapy will not alter, wherever the operation is sited, the patient's willingness to co-operate, need for analgesia, ability to move with greater or less discomfort, etc., can be anticipated from a prior knowledge of the surgical procedure he or she has undergone.

Some points to note on postoperative management

NASOGASTRIC TUBES

Any operation in which the bowel is handled may lead to a temporary paralysis of the bowel. The gastro-intestinal tract secretes eight litres of fluid each day which normally pass along the bowel and are reabsorbed. So, even if the patient is not eating or drinking, a large quantity of fluid can accumulate in the paralysed bowel and is lost to the body. Treatment is by passing a nasogastric tube and aspirating the contents of the bowel, while replacing the normal fluid and electrolyte requirements of the body intravenously.

An alternative, though less common method of keeping the stomach empty is to pass a gastrostomy tube directly through the anterior abdominal wall into the stomach at the time of the operation.

Nasogastric tubes are usually left unspigotted and thus drain freely into a narrow disposable polythene bag about 1 inch × 14 inches (2·5 × 35·5 cm). Even if the patient has been aspirated immediately prior to physiotherapy, change of position will suddenly produce a great deal of fluid which will collect in the bag at best, or leak all over the bed at worst. The physiotherapist should never become so absorbed in treating the patient's chest that she fails to check the nasogastric situation frequently. She will be ill repaid for a moment's carelessness. It is quite sufficient to empty the bag in time, as often as necessary, and report the total amount to the nurse in charge of the patient's fluid balance. The patient should not be aspirated without first seeking permission from the nursing staff. It may be that the frequency of aspiration has been decreased to two or even four hourly treatments in an effort to build up the patient's absorption tolerance.

N.B. Nasogastric tubes can usually be passed or repassed in the ward *except* after oesophageal surgery where this may be very dangerous. It is, therefore, most important that nasogastric tubes should not be accidentally removed after surgery to the oesophagus.

DRAINS

These are frequently used after major surgery. Their purpose is to drain body fluids to the surface or to allow pus, that would otherwise form an abscess, to be discharged. Drains are fixed in position with a suture, and, except in the case of long drains, a safety pin is pinned through the drain to prevent it slipping into the abdomen. Sometimes drains are attached to a vacuum flask (Redivac) so that fluids may be sucked out, or occasionally to a mechanical sucker. Following thoracotomy an underwater seal drain is used to allow air as well as fluid to be expelled from the pleural cavity, allowing the lung to re-expand. Obviously tubes of this type must be clamped before either of the bottles are elevated.

Apart from ascertaining exactly which type and where any drainage tubes are before commencing treatment, the physiotherapist must disregard them as far as is possible. There is always sufficient length to permit normal movement and physiotherapy to be performed with safety. She must also encourage the patient to do the same. Many patients are frightened by drains and are too scared to ask for the reassurance they need, and consequently lie as still as possible.

CATHETERS

These are of course a form of drain. Indwelling catheters are frequently left in the bladder following pelvic operations and almost always following operations on the genito-urinary system. They are held in position by a balloon which may be blown up once the catheter is in the bladder, and they are usually connected to a closed drainage system so that bacteria are excluded from the urinary tract. Sometimes there is a bifurcation in the catheter leading to a washout set so that the bladder can be irrigated following surgery to prevent a build-up of blood clots. A catheter is usually fixed lightly to the upper thigh and frequently the patient needs encouragement to move this leg as much as the other one.

ABDOMINAL SURGERY

UPPER GASTRO-INTESTINAL OPERATIONS

Most operations on the upper gastro-intestinal tract, that is to say the oesophagus, stomach and duodenum, are done for peptic ulceration or for cancer.

Oesophago-gastrectomy

This operation, carried out through a thoraco-abdominal incision, is performed where a radical resection of cancer of the lower end of the oesophagus or the upper part of the stomach is possible.

POSTOPERATIVE PHYSIOTHERAPY

This will follow a normal thoracotomy pattern as described under thoracic surgery (see Chapter 9 of *Chest, Heart and Vascular Disorders for Physiotherapists*). The physiotherapist will be faced with the added problems of an incision extended into the abdomen, the almost certainly very sick and weak condition of the patient, and the fact that because he will be allowed nothing by mouth, coughing will be even more difficult than usual. This is because the mouth and throat become very dry despite frequent oral toilet performed by the nursing staff. This is possibly the most difficult postoperative condition a physiotherapist is likely to meet on a general surgical ward, and indeed the patient may well prove to be a candidate for admission to an intensive therapy unit.

Treatment will be carried out three to four times daily on the first two days, perhaps decreasing to twice daily thereafter. Supervision will be necessary until he leaves hospital. A pleural effusion often develops which may need aspirating and will certainly make it difficult to keep full expansion of the left lower lobe, the part of the lung which will have been at greatest risk since the operation. Postural drainage is usually permitted and is a valuable aid in clearing secretions from the lung base, but the surgeon must always confirm that this is allowed.

Total gastrectomy

This operation, possibly involving a thoracic incision, is performed for cancer of the body of the stomach. Since the ends of the oesophagus and duodenum cannot be readily brought together it is usual to close off the duodenal end and to bring up a loop of upper small intestine and anastomose that to the lower end of the oesophagus. The spleen and part of the pancreas may also be removed. The distal end of the duodenum will be anastomosed to the jejunum.

Partial gastrectomy

There are two types of operation—Bilroth I and Polya.

Cancer of the distal or antral end of the stomach may be treated by radical removal of the distal half or two-thirds of the stomach. The cut end of the stomach may be anastomosed directly to the duodenum (Bilroth I gastrectomy) or alternatively the duodenal end may be closed off and the stomach anastomosed to a loop of small intestine (Polya gastrectomy).

Gastric and duodenal ulcer may also be treated by Polya or Bilroth I gastrectomy.

POSTOPERATIVE PHYSIOTHERAPY

The main point to stress here is that it is essential that routine treatment is carried out at least twice daily for at least three days. It is simply essential to roll the patient from side to side and, frequently, rolling with tipping will be desirable. Analgesia will always be necessary so that the times of physiotherapy must be arranged to follow injections by at least 20 to 30 minutes. Upper abdominal operations make it very hard to move the diaphragm and thus the lower lobes of the lungs without discomfort, and the physiotherapist may meet a situation perhaps following an emergency operation where the patient has realized that if he stays quite still he is relatively pain-free, and thus he may not have taken a deep breath for hours. Much valuable ground will have been lost. The advantages of teaching pre-operatively will be obvious.

Vagotomy and pyloroplasty

This is a lesser operation much to be preferred for most cases of duodenal ulcer and some cases of gastric ulcer.

Duodenal ulcer is caused by increase in the stomach acid. Division of the nerves which excite acid secretion (vagotomy) cuts down the acid production in the stomach and allows the ulcer to heal. However, since vagotomy also reduces gastric contraction a larger exit from the stomach has to be made (pyloroplasty) to allow the stomach to empty properly. A new operation, 'highly selective vagotomy', is being assessed. The aim of the operation is to cut down the acid production of the stomach without interfering with the ability of the stomach to contract so that a pyloroplasty becomes unnecessary.

POSTOPERATIVE PHYSIOTHERAPY
This is routine.

Laparotomy

When this is performed for cancer of the oesophagus or stomach which has become so advanced that it is irremovable, there are three possibilities.

(*i*) If the growth is in the oesophagus or upper part of the stomach, a rigid tube may be passed upwards through it to allow the uninterrupted passage of fluids and soft food.

(*ii*) If the growth is in the lower part of the stomach a loop of small bowel may be brought up and anastomosed to the upper part of the stomach, thus allowing food to bypass the growth (gastro-jejunostomy or gastro-enterostomy).

(*iii*) Nothing at all may be possible (laparotomy and closure).

POSTOPERATIVE PHYSIOTHERAPY
This must often of necessity be a very modified routine since at best the patient is weak, frail, anaemic and has been half-starved, and if he is also bronchitic, is in no state to tolerate sufficient physiotherapy at any session to clear his chest. At worst the prognosis may be a matter of a week or two, or perhaps a few days. This is where close liaison with the nursing and medical staff is essential, so that the policy regarding the patient is known to the physiotherapist and the amount of physiotherapy to be given is known to the rest of the team. Usually a compromise is made whereby the physiotherapist is at hand to assist in clearing the chest if this will help to keep the patient more comfortable, but will be prepared to omit a treatment if the patient is resting comfortably. Obviously all that has been said about analgesia applies with special poignancy here.

Repair of hiatus hernia

This operation may be done either from above, through the chest, or alternatively through the abdomen. Hiatus hernia is a common condition where the stomach, which normally lies within the abdominal cavity, is pushed up through the oesophageal hiatus into the chest. Usually the symptoms can be controlled without operation but in a few patients operation is necessary.

POSTOPERATIVE PHYSIOTHERAPY
This is as for a routine thoracotomy or a routine upper abdominal incision, except that the patient must never be tipped or tilted below the horizontal without the surgeon's knowledge and consent. Usually this will be given after 24 to 48 hours. But the pressure which tilting might put on a newly repaired diaphragm is not for a physiotherapist to decide.

BILIARY OPERATIONS

Cholecystectomy

This is the commonest operation performed on patients with gallstones. These stones cause pain and inflammation of the gall-bladder in which they are formed. A high proportion of patients are obese and it is essential that an adequate exposure is made. The incision is often Kocher's Subcostal. Beginning in the mid-line below the xiphoid process, it runs one inch (2.5 cm) below and parallel to the costal margin. It may, however, be an upper right paramedian incision.

POSTOPERATIVE PHYSIOTHERAPY
From the above it will be realized that the right lower lobe is greatly at risk. This is a painful operation and the patient even when co-operative may find great difficulty in maintaining full expansion of the right lung. Analgesia, followed by rolling especially onto the left side with localized deep breathing against gentle resistance is of the greatest importance. It is often not the quantity of secretions but the presence of quite a small plug of mucus blocking a part of the right lower lobe which is responsible for chest complications. Tipping is sometimes of value. Adequate careful pre-operative instruction cannot be stressed too

highly. Treatment will be needed for at least one week. Often it is safer to supervise until discharge from hospital in ten to fourteen days.

Exploration of common bile duct

When a stone has escaped from the gall-bladder into the common bile duct, impeding the flow of bile from the liver into the duodenum and causing jaundice, this operation is performed, the duct is explored and the stone removed. A 'T'-tube is usually left in the common bile duct to allow bile to flow to the surface while the inflammation in the bile duct settles down. These T-tubes can be safely removed at ten to twelve days. If the lower end of the common bile duct is narrowed it may either be widened (sphincteroplasty) or alternatively another opening can be made between the bile duct and the duodenum (chole-dochoduodenostomy).

POSTOPERATIVE PHYSIOTHERAPY
This is even more difficult to treat than cholecystectomy as the anaesthetic will have lasted longer and the T-tube is more uncomfortable than a simple drain.

Cholecystojejunostomy

This is performed when the cause of jaundice is carcinoma of the head of the pancreas. Usually this is advanced by the time the diagnosis is made and all that can be done is to provide relief of the jaundice by this operation, which joins a loop of the small bowel to the gall-bladder, thus bypassing the obstruction at the lower end of the bile duct.

POSTOPERATIVE PHYSIOTHERAPY
This is modified due to the frail condition of the patient and an extremely poor prognosis. Especial care is needed with leg exercises, as the patient can sometimes be mobilized and spend a short period at home.

Whipple's operation

This is a very major operation involving removal of part of the stomach, duodenum, pancreas and lower end of the common bile duct. It is performed for a small carcinoma of the head of the pancreas or the bile duct.

The patient is usually to be found on intensive therapy for two or three days, often rolling is restricted and the patient is nursed mainly lying on the back. Treatment must be discussed with the surgeon in charge.

LOWER ABDOMINAL SURGERY

OPERATIONS ON THE LARGE AND SMALL INTESTINES

Appendicectomy
This is the commonest surgical emergency and the commonest operation. It is usually performed through a right grid-iron incision.

POSTOPERATIVE PHYSIOTHERAPY
This is variable, all patients should be checked and have routine physiotherapy until they are fully mobile and have normal temperatures. This can be in one or two days in the case of children or non-smoking adults. The physiotherapist should be prepared for major treatment two or three times daily for several days, in the case of heavy smokers, bronchitics, patients admitted with a heavy cold, or in those with potential wound infection or pelvic sepsis due to perforation of the appendix. In the elderly (65 and upwards) appendicitis can prove fatal unless great care and skill are available.

Resection of part of the small intestine

A length of small bowel sometimes has to be removed because it contains an area of inflammation or a tumour or because its blood supply has been impaired by an embolus or from a strangulated hernia. The ends of bowel will be joined up directly.

Partial colectomy

A length of large intestine frequently has to be removed because it contains a tumour, an area of inflammation such as diverticulitis,

Crohn's disease, or ulcerative colitis. In most cases the ends of bowel can be joined up directly, but occasionally this is unsafe and the ends of bowel have to be brought out onto the surface of the abdomen where the stool may be passed into a bag. This opening is called a colostomy and will probably only be temporary, being closed at a later date.

Anterior resection of rectum

Sometimes the disease requiring resection is high in the rectum and resection is possible without removing the anus. These patients may have a colostomy, usually only temporarily.

Abdominoperineal resection of rectum

This is a very major operation performed where the disease requiring resection lies very close to the anus, and in order to make sure of a cure the whole rectum and the anus as well must be removed. In these patients a permanent colostomy has to be made.

Total colectomy with formation of ileostomy

This is performed for some patients with ulcerative colitis or with Crohn's disease (regional ileitis). The whole colon is removed and the cut end of small bowel is brought to the surface forming an ileostomy which is obviously permanent. The rectum and anus are often removed as well as the whole colon and this can be referred to as a *pan-procto total colectomy*. These patients are frequently young adults. They are often gravely ill pre-operatively, weighing three or four stone (19–25 kg) less than their normal weight, and the improvement within weeks of the operation to remove the diseased colon is often dramatic.

The ability of a patient to accept and manage a colostomy or ileostomy varies enormously but many patients, apart from a few minor alterations to their daily routine, are able to live near normal lives once they have learnt to manage their own appliance. Great help and support is available from the Colostomy Welfare group and from members of the Ileostomy Association, themselves fellow sufferers who have overcome their own difficulties and gladly pass on help and useful first-hand ideas. Many hospitals now have a *stoma therapist*, usually though not always an S.R.N., whose job is specifically to meet each stoma patient, to help, encourage, and ensure that the best possible appliance is ordered for each individual. Personal contact of this type goes a long way in helping a patient through the mental and physical trauma of this type of operation. The physiotherapist should always be acquainted with the stoma therapist and her work in general, and thus perhaps during physiotherapy treatment be able to play her part in the rehabilitation by answering inevitable questions sensibly.

POSTOPERATIVE PHYSIOTHERAPY

For operations on the large and small bowel treatment will obviously vary, but on the whole, chest complications are far fewer than with upper abdominal operations, as even when there is postoperative pain it rarely affects the patient's ability to breathe deeply. Treatment should follow a normal routine. Special attention must be paid to leg exercises, as patients are often disinclined or frightened to move the knees and hips. In the case of ileostomy patients much muscle power has often to be made up before they can be fully mobilized.

HAEMORRHOIDECTOMY

This is an excision of the dilated veins of the anus, known as haemorrhoids (piles), which cause bleeding and extreme discomfort especially on defaecation. Small piles may sometimes be treated by injection, but more severe cases or prolapsed or thrombosed haemorrhoids are usually removed.

POSTOPERATIVE PHYSIOTHERAPY

This is entirely routine but it should be remembered that although the patient's abdominal wall is intact he will still experience considerable pain on coughing, and consequently can become a major problem for the physiotherapist especially if the patient is a heavy smoker.

REPAIR OF HERNIAS

A hernia is a weakness in the body wall through which the contents of the body cavity may protrude. The commonest are inguinal and femoral, both of which lie in the groin. The hernias are repaired by excising the inner lining of the hernia, the hernial sac, and strengthening the abdominal wall with sutures. Other types of hernias seen are umbilical and incisional, the latter occurring through a previous incision, usually midline, where almost always healing was delayed.

Strangulated hernia

This is a serious surgical emergency. If the neck of the hernial sac is very narrow, the contents of the hernia may become trapped and even damaged as a result of impairment of the blood supply. This is a strangulated hernia. Not infrequently the bowel, caught in the hernia, may be so damaged as to need a resection because there is intestinal obstruction.

PHYSIOTHERAPY

Although quite routine, the treatment of repaired hernias can provide a good deal of work. Heavy smokers with a pre-existing productive cough should have intensive tipping and percussion from the first postoperative day until the (almost) inevitable pyrexia settles down. Coughing is extremely uncomfortable as the abdominal muscles are involved. The patient is unlikely to be written up for very strong analgesics and often great powers of persuasion will be required from the physiotherapist before the patient will co-operate and clear his chest.

PARTIAL THYROIDECTOMY

This operation is frequently the method of choice in treating goitre or thyrotoxicosis.

An enlarged thyroid is called a goitre. This can give rise to local problems such as difficulty in swallowing or breathing or alteration in the voice.

An over-active thyroid causes thyrotoxicosis.

The operation is carried out through a collar incision low in the neck. Sutures, or more usually clips, are removed as soon as possible, probably half on the first postoperative day and the rest on the second or third day in order to give a satisfactory scar.

Very occasionally bleeding into the neck can occur following thyroidectomy, the blood clot compresses the trachea and the patient may become asphyxiated. It is then a matter of great urgency to remove all sutures both superficial and deep until a large quantity of clot is evacuated and the patient is able to breathe again.

POSTOPERATIVE PHYSIOTHERAPY

This is routine except that even non-smoking, basically non-chesty patients almost invariably produce quantities of loose, thin, mucoid sputum. Often with a sore throat and consequent reluctance to cough properly, they can become very agitated and congested. Vibrations over the sternum timed with short sharp expiratory breaths are usually most effective, but reassurance plays a large part. The occasional thyroid patient with chronic cough can become quite a chest problem and will need intensive physiotherapy. Thyroid patients make very rapid progress and by the fourth or fifth day little is needed except to supervise neck movements.

BREAST SURGERY

Most breast swellings are removed since a diagnosis of cancer of the breast can only be excluded by histological examination.

Removal of lump in the breast

This is performed usually combined with a pathological examination, known as a *frozen section*, during the operation. If the lump is benign only the lump is removed, a small corrugated drain is left in place and the patient will probably leave hospital in one or two days. She should have no alteration in her range of shoulder movements at all.

Partial mastectomy

This is a local excision of tissue performed when the lesion is definitely not malignant such as a fibro-adenoma, a simple encapsulated tumour, cysts of the breast, or for a papilloma of the duct system.

Simple mastectomy

This operation involves removal of the breast only; no muscle tissue or nodes are removed. It may be done for extensive fibrocystic disease (benign) but is the commonest operation now for malignant disease. It is frequently followed by radiotherapy to the axillary nodes when performed for malignancy. One or two drains are usually present for up to three or four days and the patient probably will not regain her pre-operative range of shoulder movement until after these are removed.

Exercises are performed from the first postoperative day to assist in maintaining shoulder movement.

Extended mastectomy (Patey)

The same incision is used as for a simple mastectomy, but the axillary nodes are removed as well. Again all muscle tissue is left intact. Radiotherapy is given following surgery. Arm exercises are performed as before.

Radical mastectomy

This operation is mentioned here as, although very seldom performed nowadays, it is still possible that the physiotherapist will meet the results of previous surgery.

It involved the excision of the breast, the entire system of lymphatic glands in the axilla, together with the ducts which connect them with the breast, the axillary fat in which these lie, and the pectoral muscles and fascia.

A very extensive incision was made for this operation in the form of an ellipse extending from just above the axilla to just below the xiphoid process of the sternum.

Chronic oedema of the arm was frequently the result. Various physical treatments were tried including elevation, massage, exercise, faradism under pressure, perhaps with a little relief, but seldom any lasting effect as the drainage system of the arm had been removed.

Postoperative arm exercises were usually started early with the surgeon's permission and little lasting loss of range resulted.

VARICOSE VEINS

Operations usually vary with the type and severity of the symptoms. Many people have varicose veins and some are treated very successfully by injections followed by accurate padding and bandaging, often as an out-patient. For a large number of patients, however, operation becomes necessary.

Ligations

These consist of mutiple small incisions to allow tying off of the tortuous veins.

Stripping

Stripping involves incisions at groin and ankle through which the veins can be removed.

Almost all patients are mobilized early, wearing effective lateral support usually in the form of bandages. These may be elastic or crepe bandages, tube grip or elastic stockings. These patients are encouraged to be up and walking on the first postoperative day.

PHYSIOTHERAPY

This is always given. Non-weight bearing, simple leg exercises, preferably having been taught pre-operatively, are supervised and encouraged on the first day, followed by re-education of walking. The patient should walk, or should sit with the legs elevated. Standing still is always to be avoided. A very small group of patients, usually those with a varicose ulcer, may remain on bed-rest for up to a week postoperatively, but it is rare even for these patients to be forbidden frequent leg exercises. Usually these are encouraged in the normal way. Only where the field of skin grafting is entered will the physiotherapist need to find out the specific requirements of the surgical team in relation to the particular case involved.

UROLOGICAL SURGERY

Endoscopic examinations

These are common to almost all patients whose urinary tract symptoms are needing full investigations.

Cystoscopy

This is the diagnostic examination of the urinary bladder.

Urethroscopy or panendoscopy

This is the examination of the urethra with an endoscope. It is also possible through an endoscope to add several other procedures to the basic examination. The commonest is biopsy, removal of a small piece of tissue for histology.

Retrograde pyelogram

This is the injection of a radio-opaque dye through a ureteric catheter into the kidney to outline the drainage system.

Cystodiathermy

This is the burning off of small benign wartlike growths (papilloma) or early bladder tumours.

It is also possible using endoscopes to resect bladder tumours, remove some (though not all) stones from the bladder and ureter and remove part of an enlarged prostate (trans-urethral resection).

PHYSIOTHERAPY
In these patients physiotherapy ranges from almost nothing, to vigorous pre-operative treatment where these examinations reveal that further major surgery will be necessary, or to routine postoperative care when the procedure has been all the patient will need to undergo to improve his symptoms.

OPERATIONS ON THE KIDNEY

Nephrectomy

Removal of a kidney will be necessary for five main groups of disease:
   (*i*) malignant tumours;
   (*ii*) pyonephrosis—gross infection of the kidney;
   (*iii*) renal tuberculosis;
   (*iv*) sometimes renal stones;
   (*v*) hydronephrosis. This is dilation of the renal pelvis due to obstruction, leading to atrophy of the kidney tissue and impaired renal function.
Always providing the remaining kidney is healthy, nephrectomy is performed. The incision is usually an oblique lumbar one through the twelfth rib bed, but it can be lower (trans-peritoneal), or occasionally higher (trans-thoracic) through the bed of the tenth rib. A drainage tube will always be present postoperatively.

Partial nephrectomy

This operation is performed where damage is more localized or where renal calculi are confined to the upper or lower parts of the kidneys.

A drainage tube will be present and also a urethral catheter to prevent or control clotting of blood in the bladder resulting from bleeding in the kidney.

Nephrolithotomy

This is an operation to remove a stone or stones from the kidney. Approach is similar to that of a nephrectomy. The organ is mobilized and an incision is made to expose the stone. Once more a drainage tube and urethral catheter are inserted.

Pyelolithotomy

This is removal of a stone from the renal pelvis.

Pyeloplasty

This is an operation to refashion the pelvis of the kidney, particularly for hydronephrosis. The obstruction causing hydronephrosis will frequently be found in the pelvic-ureteric junction and be congenital, though it can be acquired.

PHYSIOTHERAPY

In all operations on the kidney physiotherapy is most important.

Although it can be classed as routine it is here that really full and careful pre-operative training in breathing exercises, rolling from side to side and training to cough as described earlier (Chapter 1) will be proved worthwhile. These operations restrict breathing to a very great extent on the side of the operation, because the incision is large and painful with a drainage tube in place. They also restrict it on the opposite side because the patient will have been lying on this side during the operation. Analgesic cover for physiotherapy is of the greatest importance. The patient should be treated at least twice daily for the first two to three days.

Many of these patients benefit from simple trunk exercises commenced from about the fifth day. Posture correction is needed and a simple easily progressed scheme of abdominal wall exercises should accompany the patient to home or convalescence.

OPERATIONS ON THE URETER

The ureter is a tube conveying urine from the renal pelvis to the bladder. It is approximately 30 cm long and up to 1 cm in diameter.

Surgical procedures are carried out when:

(*i*) a stone is impacted in the ureter and simple endoscopic measures have failed to move it;

(*ii*) a stricture (narrowing or complete occlusion) is present;

(*iii*) a neoplasm is present which necessitates removal of the bladder and transplantation of the ureter.

Ureterolithotomy

This is an operation to remove a stone from the ureter. It is necessary especially when the stone is causing dilation of the ureter and renal pelvis with the threat of hydronephrosis, or when infection is present, or simply if it is increasing in size while stuck in the same place.

The incision selected depends on the position of the stone revealed by X-rays taken immediately pre-operatively. It does not involve opening the peritoneum. The peritoneum is retracted allowing access to the ureter at the bifurcation of the iliac vessels. The stone is then removed and a catheter inserted to confirm that no obstruction remains. A drainage tube will be present.

Ureterocolic anastomosis

This procedure is used when the bladder is removed or when an inoperable growth in the bladder makes some palliative measure necessary.

A lower mid-line incision provides access to the ureters and sigmoid colon, the ureters are mobilized and inserted into the sigmoid colon and anastomosed. Approximately one inch (2·5 cm) of ureter is buried in the wall of the sigmoid colon which provides the valvular action necessary to prevent ascending infection reaching the kidney.

POSTOPERATIVE PHYSIOTHERAPY

In these patients this is usually routine, but the physiotherapist should be aware of the profound effect such an operation must inevitably have on the morale of an already seriously ill patient. She must always be ready to help and support both the patient and the nursing staff in their efforts to come to terms, practically and mentally, with this most distressing situation. There will be a drainage tube from the anus conveying urine and mixed faecal matter at first, but the problems start after this tube is removed in about three days. Bedpans are offered every two hours day and night, and as the patient gains some control he can usually manage to hold the contents of the rectum for four hours.

Early mobilization is necessary and these patients require particular help to regain the strength in their legs. Obviously once they can reach the toilet or commode alone they feel slightly more independent.

Formation of an ileal conduit

This is an operation in which the surgeon converts a 6–8 inch (15–20 cm) segment of the ileum into a conduit or pipeline for urinary drainage. The remaining ileum is closed in end-to-end anastomosis. The conduit segment is completely isolated from the intestinal tract but with its own blood supply. One end is closed and the two ureters are inserted here; the other end is brought out through the abdominal wall forming a stoma.

This operation used to be called an ileal bladder because it was hoped that the ileal tube would act as a substitute bladder. It does not. Voluntary control is not possible and the stoma discharges a few drops of urine every 10 to 20 seconds.

The operation is performed for chronic incontinence as in some neurological conditions, or sometimes instead of a ureterocolic anastomosis in carcinoma of the bladder. It will also be found in children after, for example, irreparable damage to the urethra following a fractured pelvis and in spina bifida.

Cystectomy

Removal of the bladder may be total or partial, and is carried out for malignant disease of the bladder. Either an ileal conduit operation or ureterocolic anastomosis will be performed as described above.

OPERATIONS FOR REMOVAL OF THE PROSTATE GLAND

There are several causes of prostatic disease and the choice of procedure depends largely on the cause and the general condition and age of the patient.

The prostate is formed by glandular tissue surrounded by a capsule encircling the urethra. There are three lobes, two lateral and a middle, and 10 to 15 ducts emptying into the urethra.

Benign senile enlargement

This is very common in older men. The prostate becomes adenomatous, enlarging and closing the prostatic urethra. The capsule is also affected but it is possible to enucleate (shell out) the gland. If the patient's condition allows, an open operation will be performed.

Fibrous enlargement

This is usually caused by prostatitis. The gland remains its normal size or even smaller and it is difficult to enucleate. Endoscopic resection will be usual.

Carcinoma of the prostate

The tumour progresses, involving the surrounding tissue, fixing the gland in position and making enucleation difficult. Usually transurethral resection will be used.

Transvesical prostatectomy

In the operation a transverse suprapubic incision is made, two fingerbreadths above the pubis, and the bladder opened. The prostate is then enucleated. Some haemorrhage will occur and must be controlled by packs and diathermy. The bladder neck forms a shelf overhanging the prostatic cavity and if left could cause postoperative obstruction. A wedge of the tissue is therefore removed. A urethral catheter is then inserted with provision for bladder irrigation to prevent clot formation. A drainage tube will also be in place in case of a leak from the sutured bladder. Sometimes a vasectomy is also performed to prevent infection from the prostatic cavity descending to the epididymis.

Retropubic prostatectomy

In this operation the prostate is removed from behind the pubis but in front of the bladder. A transverse incision is made just above the pubis, which provides a view of the prostatic capsule lying anterior to the bladder. The gland is enucleated as in the transvesical approach.

Endoscopic (trans-urethral) resection of prostate

This is performed by a special optical cutting instrument being passed into the urethra. It combines the resection with control of bleeding by diathermy. Under direct vision the surgeon is able to resect the obstructing tissue gradually. Drainage via urethral catheter is routine. Provision for bladder irrigation is needed.

PHYSIOTHERAPY

Following prostatic operations physiotherapy will obviously vary and will depend on whether the patient has an abdominal incision (retropubic or transvesical) or whether he has had a trans-urethral resection only. Frequency and intensity of treatment will also be affected by the general condition of the patient pre-operatively. An elderly chronic bronchitic with an abdominal wound, drainage tube and a catheter strapped to one leg can be a very immovable person, and will require much help and persuasion to clear his chest and move his legs adequately. The difficulty should never be underestimated.

Suprapubic cystotomy

This is a direct opening into the bladder for urinary drainage purposes. It is performed when for some reason it is not possible to pass a urethral catheter, as for example, in cases of acute retention of urine or where patients are old and unable to stand a major procedure such as prostatectomy. It will also be seen following traumatic rupture of the urethra, often in quite young men.

OPERATIONS ON THE URETHRA

These are usually required for certain acquired conditions, for example rupture due to trauma such as falling astride a ladder; a crush injury from a fractured pelvis; stricture due to inflammation; and for congenital conditions such as hypospadias when the urethra opens onto the under-surface of the penis, or epispadias when the urethra opens onto the dorsum of the penis.

Ruptured urethra

If it is impossible to pass a urethral catheter, a suprapubic cystotomy is performed to divert the flow of urine. After this the extent of the damage is usually investigated, any clot or haematoma is removed and a catheter inserted for about ten days until healing is complete. Usually a repair is not attempted at this stage. *Urethroplasty* will be performed if the urethra is still not patent. This is plastic surgery using skin to construct the urethra. It is often necessary to perform the operation in two stages separated by several months. After the first stage the patient may have an opening into the perineum at the base of the penis, but at least no catheter or suprapubic drain. After the second stage normality is achieved.

Dilation of urethra

Periodic dilation may be necessary in cases as described above or where there is narrowing following inflammation.

PHYSIOTHERAPY

Following urethral operations physiotherapy is entirely routine and usually minimal, bearing in mind, however, that if the urethra has been damaged by a pelvic injury there may be the complication of a fractured pelvis to consider and treat.

ARTERIAL SURGERY

The commonest arterial disease, and the one most usually presenting a surgical problem, is arteriosclerosis. This is a degenerative disease of arteries which causes narrowing or blocking of the vessels. If a major artery becomes blocked in this way, then the blood supply to the part which it supplies becomes impaired and the viability of the part itself is threatened.

If the block is localized it may be removed (endarterectomy), or alternatively a vein or a tube of synthetic material such as Dacron may be used to bypass the block. Sometimes division of the sympathetic nerves to the legs (lumbar sympathectomy) may allow the small vessels in the leg to dilate sufficiently to produce a significant clinical improvement.

When direct arterial surgery is not possible, and the limb is causing considerable pain or is frankly gangrenous, amputation is indicated (see Chapter 12). The site of the amputation may be above, through or below the knee in these patients. The decision as to what level to amputate must take into account not only the patient's ability to manage a prosthesis, but must allow adequate blood supply to ensure healing of the stump.

Sometimes the arterial wall becomes so weak that the artery itself is dilated by the blood pressure within it. If this occurs over a limited segment an aneurysm is formed. This most commonly occurs in a major vessel such as the aorta. Occasionally as the aneurysm gets larger the wall becomes so weak that it ruptures. Prompt action with replacement of the aneurysm with a Dacron graft is a life-saving though major operation. (For further details see Chapter 18 of *Chest, Heart and Vascular Disorders for Physiotherapists*.)

CHAPTER 3

Gynaecological Conditions

by SHEILA HARRISON, MCSP

The term Gynaecology is derived from the Greek words, *gynae* = a woman and *logos* = a discourse, study or science. Thus gynaecology is the study of the woman as a whole.

It is important to bear in mind that the activity of the genital organs is controlled by the endocrine system, which itself is often influenced by the psyche (mind).

While the symptoms of many diseases are psychosomatic, the mind plays a particularly important role in gynaecological conditions. There is a great deal of fear, anxiety and embarrassment associated with these conditions and their treatment. It is important that we treat the patient with sensitivity and understanding, thinking of each as a complete person.

The physiotherapist will meet gynaecological patients in a ward situation and as out-patients.

Some understanding of the female pelvis and its contents is essential. The points of special importance for her work are the relationship of one organ to another within the pelvis and the pelvic floor muscles.

ANATOMICAL RELATIONS IN THE PELVIS

The uterus
The uterus lies in the pelvis with the bladder in front and the rectum behind (Fig. 3/1). It is tilted forward making an angle of 90° to the vagina. Its anterior and posterior surfaces are covered by peritoneum. On each side of the uterus the two layers of peritoneum meet to form the broad ligaments which then attach to the lateral walls of the pelvis.

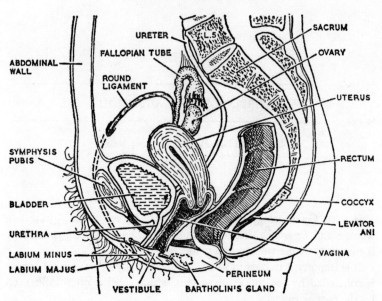

Fig. 3/1 The position and relations of the uterus.

Between the two layers run the round ligaments (round muscles) which eventually enter the deep inguinal ring, pass through the inguinal canal and finally blend with the areolar tissue of the labia majora, thus

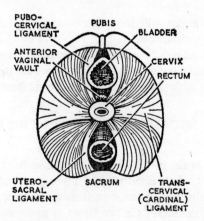

Fig. 3/2 The 'ligaments' of the cervix.

72

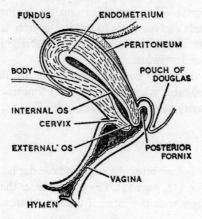

Fig. 3/3 Coronal section of the uterus.

probably helping to hold the uterus in the anteverted position. The cervix and fornices of the vagina are further supported by the cervical ligaments as shown in Fig. 3/2.

The uterus is a hollow pear-shaped organ whose narrow lower end

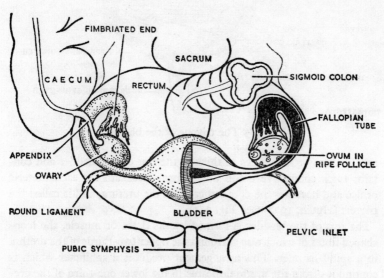

Fig. 3/4 Diagram showing the fallopian tubes.

73

is termed the cervix. This protrudes into the vagina, a canal which extends downwards and forwards to end in the vestibule (cleft between labia minora) (see Fig. 3/3). The mucous membrane lining the uterus is known as the endometrium.

Opening into the upper angles of the uterus are the right and left fallopian (uterine) tubes whose other ends are fimbriated and open into the peritoneal cavity close to the ovaries (see Fig. 3/4).

The bladder

The bladder is a hollow muscular organ whose flat base lies parallel to the vagina (see Fig. 3/1, page 72). The ureters enter the base at an angle and form a triangle with the internal urinary meatus. This triangular

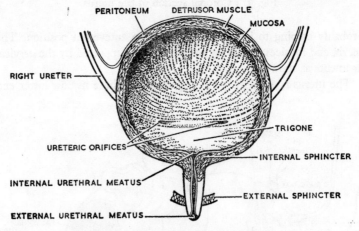

Fig. 3/5 The trigone of the bladder.

area is three or four times as thick as the rest of the bladder and contains thick connective tissue which forms a sheath for each ureteric orifice and becomes the core structure of the urethra, and is called the trigone (Hutch, 1972) (see Fig. 3/5).

The rest of the bladder is formed by the detrusor muscle, the loop-shaped fibres of which also surround the upper two-thirds of the urethra in a spiral manner. This arrangement produces a sphincter which is continuous from the urethral meatus to the lower one-third of the urethra. At this point the striated muscle fibres reflected up from the urogenital diaphragm (see Figs. 3/8, 3/9, both on page 77) form the external sphincter, the function of which is to stop, voluntarily, the urinary stream.

It will be seen from Fig. 3/6 that the urethra leaves the flat base of the bladder almost at a right angle, thus forming the anterior and posterior urethrovesical angles. These angles are lost during micturition as funnelling of the bladder base occurs. The posterior angle is frequently missing if the anterior vaginal wall is weakened, allowing the

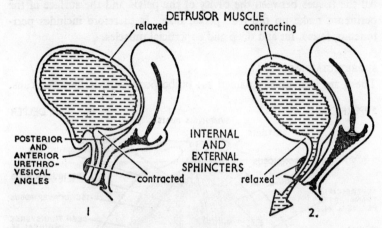

Fig. 3/6 The anterior and posterior urethrovesical angles (1) normal and (2) their disappearance during micturition.

upper part of the bladder base and the urethra to prolapse downwards and backwards (see Fig. 3/6). This is often associated with laxity of the pelvic floor muscles and results in stress incontinence (see page 89).

NERVE SUPPLY OF BLADDER

The upper part of the bladder is poorly supplied by autonomic nerve fibres while the area around the trigone is richly innervated (Llewellyn-Jones, 1972). The parasympathetic fibres are derived from S2, S3 and S4 and are motor to the detrusor muscle. The sympathetic fibres mainly derive from L1 and L2 and supply the trigone. In the voiding reflex the sensory stimuli initiated by stretch and tension in the bladder wall are carried to the sacral cord through the afferent fibres of the sacral parasympathetic nerves; the motor branch of this reflex arc is formed by the efferent fibres of these same sacral parasympathetic nerves. Although certain sensory impulses from the bladder (pain and thermal perception) are conveyed by sympathetic fibres, extensive sympathectomy does not alter bladder function. The external sphincter (voluntary) receives its nerve supply from the pudendal nerve (S2, S3, S4).

The pelvic floor

All the tissues between the cavity of the pelvis and the surface of the perineum make up the true pelvic floor. It therefore includes peritoneum, fascia, fat and deep and superficial muscles.

SUPERFICIAL MUSCLES
These are individually named as: bulbospongiosus, ischiocavernosus,

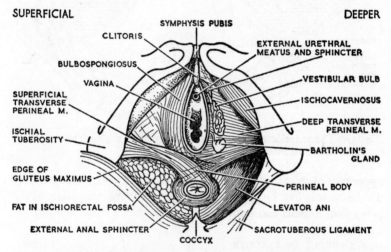

Fig. 3/7 Dissection of the perineum showing the superficial muscles.

deep and superficial transverse perineal muscles. They take origin from the ischium and pubis and are inserted into the central point of the perineum, the perineal body (see Fig. 3/7).

DEEP MUSCLES
These form the most important muscle group and together with the fascia covering their upper and lower surfaces are commonly known

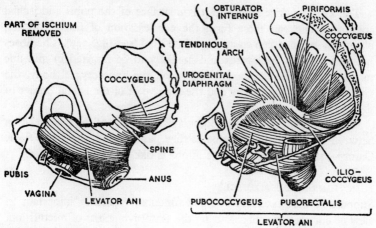

EXTERNAL VIEW   INTERNAL VIEW

Fig. 3/8 Lateral view of the pelvic diaphragm, external and internal, showing urogenital diaphragm.

as the pelvic floor muscles, though some authorities use the term 'the pelvic diaphragm' (see Fig. 3/8).

Levator ani and coccygeus form the main elements of this group and are supplied by the fourth sacral nerve. These voluntary muscles form a wide sling through which the urethra, vagina and rectum pass (Figs. 3/1, 3/8, 3/9). They also provide supporting fibres for these structures.

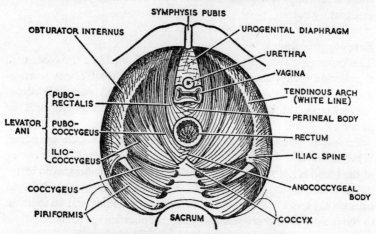

Fig. 3/9 Levator ani muscles from above.

The muscles arise from the pelvic surface of the pubis and ischial spine and between these form the condensation of fascia covering obturator internus known as the 'white line' (see Fig. 3/9). The fibres pass downwards, backwards and medially to be inserted in mid-line to the vagina, perineal body, anal canal, the anococcygeal body, the lateral border of the coccyx and the lower part of the lateral border of the sacrum.

It is important that the physiotherapist be aware of the close relation between the urethra and vagina as they pass through the pelvic floor. Damage, stretching or weakness in one is likely to affect the other.

FUNCTIONS OF DEEP MUSCLES
Support of the viscera is a prime function, especially important in view of our erect posture. During the expulsive efforts of micturition, defaecation and during parturition, the muscles are relaxed though they contract to lift the pelvic floor at the conclusion of such efforts.

They contract reflexly (unless they are very weak) when the intra-abdominal pressure is raised, e.g. when coughing or sneezing (see Stress Incontinence, page 89).

GYNAECOLOGICAL WARD

The range of conditions and operative procedures is large, so the ones most frequently found are listed on the following pages with brief explanatory notes.

Ectopic pregnancy
This occurs if a fertilized ovum becomes implanted in a site other than the uterine cavity, the fallopian tube being the most common extra-uterine site. The tubes will eventually rupture and when this occurs the operation of salpingectomy or salpingo-oophorectomy will be necessary.

Ectopic pregnancy may present as an acute or sub-acute condition. When there is a severe intraperitoneal haemorrhage and the majority of the blood is not removed during the operation, diaphragmatic irritation is often caused by the clotted blood under the diaphragm. Referred pain via C4 and C5 to the supraclavicular area results, and an increase in the incidence of postoperative chest complications is likely.

Pelvic inflammatory disease

This is an inflammatory condition of the fallopian tubes and often of the uterus secondary to bacterial infection. The infection may be primary as in tuberculosis or secondary as in gonorrhoea. Infection may also follow abortion or parturition and occasionally follows such acute inflammatory diseases as appendicitis or diverticulitis.

The disease may present as an acute attack of abdominal peritonitis which is treated by chemotherapy and occasionally by the drainage of any abscesses by the vaginal or abdominal route.

As far as physiotherapists are concerned they are more likely to meet this condition in its chronic form, when they may be requested to give a course of shortwave diathermy (see page 97). The symptoms of this chronic form of the disease are secondary dysmenorrhoea, dyspareunia and a disturbance of the menstrual pattern. Occasionally, under treatment, the condition may be exacerbated. This will be shown by the fact that the patient will be generally unwell and have an increase in her symptoms. Treatment must be stopped until the gynaecologist has been consulted.

It is worth noting that this condition is often abbreviated as P.I.D., and this may lead to confusion with the shortened form of the phrase prolapsed intervertebral disc.

Variations in the menstrual cycle

The normal cycle is defined as a blood loss lasting five days every 28 days. The range of this loss may be between one and seven days and the intervals vary between 21 and 35 days, counting from the first day of one period to the first day of the next.

There are a number of descriptive terms applied to abnormalities of the menstrual cycle.

(*i*) Amenorrhoea: the absence of menstruation. This may be primary or secondary.

(*ii*) Polymenorrhoea: too frequent periods.

(*iii*) Menorrhagia: an increase in the volume of the blood loss occurring at regular intervals. This may be an increase in the volume lost in any given time, or an increase in the duration of the loss, or both at once.

(*iv*) Intermenstrual bleeding: bleeding between periods.

(*v*) Postcoital bleeding: bleeding following coitus.

On the whole, a description of the type, frequency and character of the bleeding in simple terms is the easiest way to a clear understanding of a patient's menstrual cycle.

ABDOMINAL PAIN DUE TO NERVE ENTRAPMENT

In recent years it has been discovered that many women complaining of chronic pain in one or both iliac fossae are suffering from what has been described as the 'nerve entrapment syndrome'. These women are not suffering from gynaecological disease though they may have had gynaecological operations.

This abdominal wall pain has been described as a sharp burning pain in the abdominal wall along the outer border of the rectus sheath. The cutaneous intercostal nerves can be compressed in the posterior wall of the rectus sheath (Mehta, 1973).

Thorough investigations for evidence of serious disease will leave a small group of patients who suffer great discomfort from this condition.

Remission may be spontaneous but frequently symptoms may persist intermittently for a long time.

Diagnosis is confirmed by tensing the abdominal muscles by raising the head and shoulders from a lying position and finding the tender area, about the size of a pea. Coughing also produces the pain.

Infiltration of the tender zone with local anaesthesia relieves the symptoms temporarily and confirms the source of discomfort.

The best results are found to be from injection therapy, using an anaesthetic solution. This produces a differential block with impact on the non-myelinated and small myelinated pain fibres. Operative intervention is seldom necessary.

OPERATIONS USING A VAGINAL ROUTE

DILATATION AND CURETTAGE (D & C)
The cervix is dilated and the uterine cavity is scraped. This is used for diagnostic purposes, removal of polyps, after an incomplete abortion and as a vaginal termination of pregnancy.

SHIRODKAR SUTURE (see Fig. 3/10)
A non-absorbable suture is placed around the internal os (cervix) during early pregnancy in women whose defective cervix has dilated

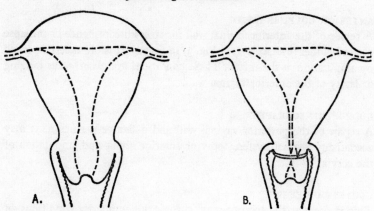

Fig. 3/10 Shirodkar suture. A. Uterus with an incompetent internal os. B. Non-absorbable suture tied round cervix at level of internal os.

prematurely in previous pregnancies, leading to late abortion (18 to 20 weeks). The suture is removed about 14 days before term. Some authorities insert this suture before pregnancy.

CONE BIOPSY
A conical segment is removed from the cervix. It is used as a diagnostic check after positive smears from a Papanicolaou test.

INCISION OF BARTHOLIN'S ABSCESS
An acute infection in the gland of the labium major which has to be incised.

EXCISION OF BARTHOLIN'S CYST
An excision of a cyst of the gland at the base of the labium major. The cyst is often due to chronic infection.

VULVECTOMY
An excision of the skin in the vulval area for skin disease including malignancy. In the presence of malignant disease it often includes the whole of the vulva and the inguinal glands.

VAGINAL HYSTERECTOMY
The removal of the uterus vaginally for menorrhagia or prolapse.

ANTERIOR COLPORRHAPHY

A repair of the anterior vaginal wall for stress incontinence or prolapse of the bladder (cystocele) (see Fig. 3/12, p. 91). It is often accompanied by amputation of the cervix. These conditions are observed as bulging or laxity of the anterior vaginal wall.

COLPOPERINEORRAPHY

A repair of the posterior vaginal wall and defective perineum. It may accompany vaginal hysterectomy or anterior repair and amputation of the cervix.

CAUTERY OF CERVIX

This is done as the treatment of chronic inflammatory conditions of the cervix, symptoms of which are an offensive discharge and dyspareunia.

INSUFFLATION OF THE FALLOPIAN TUBES

This procedure is used to check the patency of the tubes in cases of infertility. Carbon dioxide is blown into the uterus from a pressure apparatus which shows the passage of gas through the tubes on a calibrated drum (kymograph).

OPERATIONS WITH ABDOMINAL INCISIONS

Types of incision (see Fig. 3/11, p. 83)

Transverse incisions are variations of the Pfannenstiel incision and are commonly known as the 'bikini'. They are relatively bloodless and there is little chance of an incisional hernia. The patient has less postoperative discomfort than with other incisions. The disadvantages lie in its taking slightly longer to perform, and it occasionally gives inadequate exposure for large tumours.

A *mid-line* incision is a longitudinal one in which the linea alba is incised. It can be performed rapidly and is relatively bloodless due to the fibrous tissue being incised. The disadvantages are a definite danger of an incisional hernia developing later, because fibrous tissue heals less efficiently. There is generally more postoperative discomfort.

A *paramedian* incision is made to the right or left of centre and carries a low incidence of incisional hernia. It is slower to perform than a mid-line incision and is likely to produce more bleeding than mid-line or transverse incisions. Postoperative discomfort is similar to that experienced with a mid-line incision.

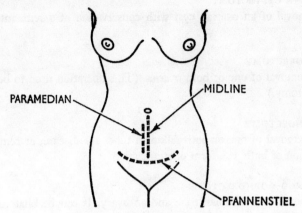

Fig. 3/11 Types of incisions.

TOTAL HYSTERECTOMY

The whole uterus is removed. Occasionally the cervix is left in situ, thus becoming a subtotal hysterectomy.

HYSTEROTOMY

A termination of pregnancy by removing the fetus and products of conception through an incision in the uterus.

WERTHEIM'S HYSTERECTOMY

The removal of the whole uterus, tubes and ovaries, upper half of the vagina, broad ligaments and the lymph nodes around the iliac vessels and the lateral pelvic walls. It is performed for carcinoma of the cervix and occasionally for carcinoma of the uterus.

MYOMECTOMY

The removal of fibroids from the uterus. It can also be done vaginally if the fibroid is being extruded as a polyp.

VENTROSUSPENSION

A correction of the position of the uterus from the retroverted to the anteverted position by shortening the round ligaments or by drawing

83

them through the peritoneum and rectus muscles and suturing them to each other in front of the rectus muscles.

OVARIAN CYSTECTOMY
A removal of an ovarian cyst with conservation of a remnant of the ovary.

OOPHORECTOMY
The removal of one or both ovaries. (This operation used to be called ovariotomy.)

SALPINGECTOMY
The removal of one or both fallopian tubes for disease, or removal of a portion of both as a form of sterilization.

SALPINGO-OOPHORECTOMY
A removal of a fallopian tube and an ovary. It can be bilateral. It is sometimes associated with hysterectomy.

BIOPSY OR WEDGE RESECTION OF THE OVARY
A diagnostic biopsy operation on the ovary for endocrine problems.

FALLOPIAN PLASTIC OPERATIONS
Restoration of patency to a blocked fallopian tube in an attempt to cure infertility.

PELVIC EXENTERATION
A radical operation for pelvic malignant disease which entails removal of the uterus, rectum or bladder or both with transplantation of ureters and colostomy.

POSTERIOR COLPOTOMY
An aspiration or drainage of the pouch of Douglas through the posterior fornix.

LAPAROSCOPY
A means of visualizing the abdominal contents after the induction of a pneumoperitoneum without making a large abdominal incision. Operative procedures can be carried out by this method, e.g. ovarian biopsy and sterilization using diathermy.

PRESACRAL NEURECTOMY

This is done for primary spasmodic dysmenorrhoea. The fibres of the presacral nerve lying in front of the first part of the sacrum are divided.

LAPAROTOMY

Opening the abdomen for investigation.

Operations for stress incontinence

VAGINAL

See under Vaginal route, p. 82 (anterior colporrhaphy).

ABDOMINAL

These are a series of abdominal or combined abdominal and vaginal operations, the principle of which is the construction of some form of sling to reform the posterior vesico-urethral angle of the bladder (see Fig. 3/6, p. 75). Such operations are named after their originators, e.g. Aldridge, Millin, Marshall-Marchetti-Krantz, and others. These may be accomplished by the insertion of artificial substances, natural transplanted tissues, or the use of contiguous tissues (vaginal). These materials are either anchored to the periosteum and ligaments of the bony pubis or the sheath of the rectus abdominis.

PHYSIOTHERAPY

Most patients in the ward will be having an operation, so the work of the physiotherapist will be similar to that on other surgical wards (Chapter 2), but with certain additions and some differences in technique.

ADDITIONS

Pelvic tilting (backwards). This encourages the viscera to move away from the incised abdominal wall, so increasing the patient's comfort. It should be taught in the crook-lying, lying, sitting and standing positions to encourage an upright posture.

Pelvic floor exercises (see page 95). These are vital because the pelvic floor needs re-education due to the condition or as a result of the surgery. The starting date must be agreed by consultation with the surgeon.

Patients who have had a pelvic operation appear to be particularly susceptible to deep vein thrombosis, therefore special precautions should be taken:

If Tubigrip or an elastic bandage has not been applied prior to operation or in the theatre, the physiotherapist may be asked to apply this when the patient returns to the ward.

The foot of the bed can be elevated and a bed cradle used to facilitate frequent foot and leg movements.

Extra emphasis should be placed on deep breathing, practised frequently, to improve venous return.

DIFFERENCES IN TECHNIQUE

Due to the frequency of the use of the Pfannenstiel incision the author has found that the best way to assist the patient with postoperative breathing and coughing is as shown in Plates 3/1 and 3/2 (between pages 160 and 161). The instructions are:

Blow out slowly and continuously until the lungs feel empty.

Shut the mouth and draw air up through the nose slowly, feeling the chest expanding. When the chest feels comfortably full start blowing out again.

After emptying and filling the lungs three or four times, a sharp command 'cough *now*' is given, while firm pressure from the patient's and physiotherapist's hands is given over the incision. If the patient has sutures in her vagina or perineum she should apply firm pressure over her sanitary pad when she coughs. This will lessen the bulging of the abdomen or perineum and greatly increase the patient's comfort and confidence.

Graduated exercises

A scheme of graduated exercises in the form of a duplicated list is very useful. Each patient can be given a list at the time she is taught preoperative breathing. A brief explanation about the list given at this time shows the patient that the breathing exercises are part of a programme of continuous care which aims to reduce the effects of the anaesthetic and the operation and speed her restoration to normality.

As well as the three exercises already mentioned above the following should be included: Strengthening exercises for the abdominal and back muscles; and Correct lifting methods.

Infra-red radiation

Heat from an infra-red source can be very effective in speeding the healing of infected and slow-healing wounds or haematomas. The dilatation of the capillaries and arterioles in the superficial tissues allows more blood to flow to the tissues, thus aiding the reaction to and clearing of the infection because more white blood cells are present. The increased metabolism in the heated area results in an increased demand for oxygen and nutrients and the output of waste products.

Care should be taken to ensure that an adequate area of skin around the incision is exposed to the heat, as thermal sensation in the proximity of a wound is frequently impaired.

Physiotherapists working in an Obstetric or Gynaecological department will find themselves in a very emotional atmosphere. This emotion may reveal itself in a coarseness and vulgarity which they may find distasteful and unbecoming to women. At the opposite extreme they will find a reticence and embarrassment that makes it difficult to achieve any satisfactory contact with the patient.

There are, however, certain repetitive phenomena which physiotherapists will meet in both specialities. These are emotional in origin and tend to occur about the third and the ninth day after delivery or a major operation.

After parturition the 'let down' and relief accompanied by discomfort in the perineum and breasts often cause depression on the third day. On the eighth or ninth day, particularly in primigravidae, the realization of the responsibility that they have now assumed weighs heavily upon them.

The same thing applies, though the reasons are somewhat different, after major gynaecological operations. The second and third post-operative days are often the most uncomfortable. At this time some patients start to show concern about the effect of the operation on their femininity. This is particularly true of a hysterectomy. On the ninth or tenth day, just prior to her discharge, the patient becomes worried about her ability to reassume her role as a complete woman and mother.

GYNAECOLOGY IN THE OUTPATIENT DEPARTMENT

Since there are many gynaecological conditions where physiotherapy is not indicated, the role of the gynaecologist is to select those patients who will benefit from the particular skills of a physiotherapist.

As some of these skills are only acquired as a result of postregistration training, it is accepted that some stages of the treatments which follow cannot be undertaken by a student. However, a student can learn much by observing an experienced physiotherapist treating a patient and assisting where appropriate.

Treatments are likely to fall into two categories: restoration of function by re-education of the pelvic floor muscles, and shortwave diathermy.

Symptoms of weak pelvic floor muscles

The pelvic floor muscles have many functions (see page 76), so a wide range of symptoms can be expected to show if the muscles are weak. The most important of these are listed below, together with the patient's descriptions of the symptoms. A patient may present with one or many of these symptoms:

Stress incontinence: leaking of urine when coughing, sneezing, laughing or running;

Cystocele and urethrocele: a bulgy lump just inside the vagina;

Pelvic floor laxity: lack of satisfaction during coitus and inability to retain a contraceptive diaphragm;

First degree prolapse: heaviness in the vagina and 'something coming down';

Frequency: passing urine very often;

Obesity: symptoms get worse as weight increases.

Each of these symptoms will be discussed individually before any treatment is described.

Incontinence

This can be divided into four types, all are non-neurogenic, i.e. they do not originate in the nervous system. They are: complete incontinence; overflow incontinence with retention; urge incontinence; and stress incontinence.

Stress incontinence is the most relevant to this text, however brief notes about the other types are included to enable the student to have a better understanding of the problem.

COMPLETE INCONTINENCE

This is due to the development of a fistula which allows urine to leak into the surrounding tissues. The rate of this flow is dependent on the size of the fistula.

The most common sites of a fistula are: (*i*) between bladder and vagina (vesicovaginal); (*ii*) between ureter and vagina (ureterovaginal); (*iii*) between urethra and vagina (urethrovaginal).

The *causes* of a fistula may be congenital or acquired. Examples of the latter include childbirth, surgery, radiotherapy, or a new growth.

Treatment: surgery.

OVERFLOW INCONTINENCE

Overflow incontinence with retention of urine is generally caused by an obstruction to the outflow of urine. This causes the bladder to fill and overflow, giving passage to small amounts of urine at frequent intervals.

Causes. Overflow incontinence with retention may be caused by a mass in the pelvis such as a retroverted gravid uterus, a fibroid or an ovarian cyst; or it may be caused by trauma to the bladder or its nerve supply during a pelvic operation or childbirth, which results in the mechanism of the micturition reflex being damaged.

Treatment. This varies with the cause. Physiotherapy is not indicated.

URGE INCONTINENCE

Urge incontinence occurs when the desire to micturate overwhelms the voluntary capacity to control bladder function, and spontaneous emptying of the bladder occurs at any time.

This is an inflammatory condition which can be acute or chronic. Infected residual urine causes irritation of the base of the bladder (the trigone) giving a basal trigonitis. This causes the micturition reflex to be released earlier than usual

Treatment: antibiotics or surgery.

Stress incontinence

This may be defined as the accidental voiding of varying amounts of urine down the urethra when the intra-abdominal pressure is raised, as in a cough or sneeze. The number of activities which produce leaking vary with the severity of the condition.

This is the most interesting type of incontinence to the physiotherapist because the choice of treatments lies between physiotherapy and surgery. Well-directed physiotherapy can so often make surgery unnecessary. Women with stress incontinence are always distressed and embarrassed by their condition. However the word 'stress' does not indicate an anxiety state but describes a sudden increase in intra-abdominal pressure resulting in the involuntary passage of urine.

CAUSES OF STRESS INCONTINENCE

These are: loss of elasticity of connective tissue of the pelvic floor; atrophy of urethral musculature leading to a decrease in urethral turgor; weakness of the deep pelvic floor muscles.

The withdrawal of hormones in menopausal women makes them particularly prone to the first two conditions. The administration of oestrogen or a combination of oestrogen and androgenic hormones relieves the condition. The loss of turgor in the urethra causes a loss of resistance to the passage of urine in the urethra and can be an important factor in incontinence.

Anabolic preparations are occasionally prescribed to aid the strengthening of the pelvic floor muscles.

Weakness of the pelvic floor muscles is almost always due to the effects of childbearing, where postnatal exercises have been omitted or ineffectively taught.

Cystocele and urethrocele

The anterior vaginal wall may prolapse independently of any uterine descent. When the upper part is involved the bladder herniates backwards due to its connection to the vagina via the pubocervical fascia (see Fig. 3/12, p. 91). A lump is formed which the patient can feel and if the condition is severe the bladder is incompletely emptied. The residual urine easily becomes infected and frequency and dysuria are then additional symptoms.

If the lower part of the anterior vaginal wall prolapses, the urethra is displaced backwards and a urethrocele develops (see Fig. 3/13, p. 91).

Causes. Prolapse may be caused by prolonged pressure by the presenting part in the second stage of labour. Damage to the urogenital diaphragm precipitates a urethrocele.

Prolapse of the posterior vaginal wall produces a rectocele.

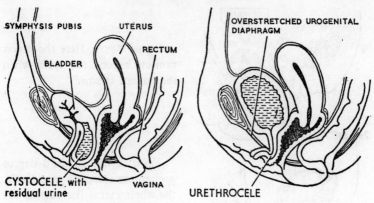

Fig. 3/12 Cystocele.   Fig. 3/13 Urethrocele.

Pelvic floor laxity

The superficial and deep muscles of the pelvic floor play an important part during sexual intercourse. Muscular insufficiency can lead to sexual problems; also difficulty in retaining a contraceptive diaphragm in the vagina.

Prolapse of the uterus

The word prolapse means 'to slip out of place'. When the uterus prolapses, the upper vagina which is attached to the uterus is drawn downwards as well.

Three degrees of uterine prolapse are recognized:

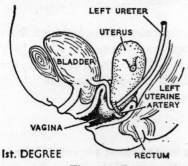

First degree. Here the uterus descends inside the vagina to, or almost to, the introitus.

Fig. 3/14 Degrees of uterovaginal prolapse.

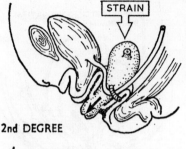

2nd DEGREE

Second degree. Here the cervix projects beyond the vulva when the patient strains.

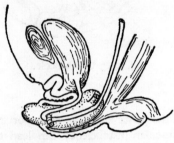

3rd DEGREE
COMPLETE PROCIDENTIA

Fig. 3/14 *continued*

Third degree. In third degree prolapse or complete procidentia, the whole uterus lies outside the vagina and most of the vagina is inside out. The cervix may become ulcerated and the acute angulation of the urethra causes difficulty in the initiation of micturition. Hydronephrosis can occasionally be present. It is interesting to note how quickly these severe changes can resolve when the prolapse is reduced. A period of bed-rest and vaginal packing generally precedes operative treatment of a procidentia (see Fig. 3/14, above).

CAUSES

Deficiency in the uterine supports predisposes to prolapse. Three main reasons for the supports to become weaker are:

Congenital;

Overstretching during childbirth, especially if the patient bears down before she is fully dilated. A prolonged second stage with a large baby will also damage the uterine supports, as will too much pressure on the fundus of the uterus when attempting to deliver the placenta;

Withdrawal of hormones at the menopause.

Frequency

The word frequency should only be used to denote a repeated desire to pass urine even when the bladder is empty. This occurs with urge

incontinence, but can frequently be met in patients with stress incontinence where their fear of leaking urine is linked subconsciously
with a desire to keep their bladder empty—so the repeated attempts to
pass urine become a habit. This could be called 'self-induced frequency',
and can be regulated by bladder training (see Stress incontinence,
p. 89).

Obesity

If the patient is overweight she has a lot of extra fat around and in
between her pelvic organs. This puts considerable extra weight and
strain on her pelvic floor, especially if she has a persistent cough.

It should be noted that local vaginal infections, such as trichomonas,
will be treated by the gynaecologist, as will involutional vaginitis
which is particularly found in menopausal women. The latter responds
readily to the administration of oestrogen.

Once a physiotherapist has a full understanding of the symptoms she
may find in a patient, she can start considering the treatment.

RESTORATION OF FUNCTION BY RE-EDUCATION
OF PELVIC FLOOR MUSCLES

Method

The treatment is in two parts, firstly the interview or assessment and
secondly the scheme of exercises. Group therapy is the ideal method as
patients gain much from contact with other women with the same problem and an element of competition enters for the overweight during
the weekly 'weigh-in'.

There will always be some patients who for reasons of distance or
temperament cannot attend a weekly session. Repeat visits at three- or
four-weekly intervals are found to be satisfactory.

INTERVIEW

The diversity of the patient's symptoms makes it essential that a physiotherapist specializing in this work conducts the interview, which forms
the assessment of the patient. Quiet, privacy and time (at least 45
minutes) are required.

Gynaecological Conditions

HISTORY

The following points should be covered.

(*i*) Parity.

(*ii*) Type of delivery. Episiotomy and the number of stitches is not important, since an episiotomy performed to enable a quicker delivery of the baby is a good obstetric practice. It is relevant to enquire about the length of the first and second stages of labour. A persistent anterior lip of the cervix or prolonged pushing are likely to produce extra stretching and weakening of ligaments and muscles of the pelvic floor. A fast second stage can be equally traumatic.

Forceps extraction does not generally produce added trauma, though a high Kielland rotation may do so.

(*iii*) What size were her babies; was polyhydramnios present?

(*iv*) Did she do postnatal exercises? Was exercise for the pelvic floor included?

(*v*) Menstrual cycle.

(*vi*) Contraception.

(*vii*) Dyspareunia? Sexual satisfaction?

(*viii*) Micturition habits. Frequency during the day or night? Does she have to change her pants often during the day? Does leaking prevent social activity? Does she wear a pad? Has she any condition that makes her cough or sneeze much? Does she smoke?

(*ix*) Any other illness, operations or accidents?

(*x*) *Explain* the anatomy of the pelvis and the pelvic floor using diagrams. Relate the patient's symptoms to her weak pelvic floor and its re-education.

VAGINAL EXAMINATION

This is only undertaken by an experienced physiotherapist.

This examination is an essential part of the treatment. It is the only way to be sure the patient is actually contracting her pelvic floor muscles.

Method. The patient lies on her left side with her knees comfortably drawn up. The physiotherapist washes her hands and puts on disposable gloves. With the thumb and index finger of her left hand she separates the labia and looks for signs of vaginal irritation. Ask the patient to cough, notice any bulging at the introitus, also any leakage of urine. Then introduce the index and middle fingers of the right hand slowly, gently, upwards and backwards. Locate fornices and cervix and check

94

the state of the vaginal walls. It is obvious that great care must be taken during this procedure, especially if the woman is nulliparous.

The examiner then withdraws her fingers until the distal two phalanges are palpating the posterior vaginal wall. Say to the patient 'Squeeze on my fingers as much as you can'. Strong deep pelvic floor muscles will nip the fingers very firmly. In this way the strength of the muscles can be estimated by the amount of contraction the patient can produce.

As the levator muscles are not visible, a closing and lifting sensation in the vagina is the only proof the patient has that the correct muscles are working.

If there is a major weakness of the pelvic floor, a contraction of the gluteus maximus can produce an irradiation overflow into the levatores (Samson Wright, 1971). This could be done as follows. 'Squeeze your seat muscles so that you close your back passage, now try to close your vagina, now increase the effort so that you draw both passages up inside.'

When the physiotherapist is satisfied that the patient has understood how to contract her pelvic floor muscles, she withdraws her fingers. The patient repeats the contraction, checking the sensation in her vagina and relating this to the one she must produce when practising at home.

Pelvic floor contractions should also be practised sitting in a chair and standing (as if at the sink or in a shop).

Finally, explain to the patient that a definite programme must be followed if this treatment is to be effective.

Programme

Four pelvic floor contractions on the hour every hour, each contraction being held for four seconds. A cake timer or alarm clock will act as a stimulus until her brain gets used to the regime.

Bladder training is necessary if she has mentioned symptoms indicating frequency. This consists of consciously lengthening the time between each attempt to pass urine and using pelvic floor contractions when it becomes difficult to hold urine.

If the patient is overweight, start reducing, using the advice of a doctor and a dietician.

If the patient has a cough the chest clinic will give advice, or if the cough is caused by smoking the number of cigarettes smoked must be

Gynaecological Conditions

reduced. Emphasis must be laid on the strain and overstretching of the pelvic floor produced by persistent coughing or sneezing. She must learn to contract her pelvic floor muscles just before she coughs or sneezes.

The patient is asked to stop and start the flow of urine three times every time she empties her bladder.

The patient joins a group, with an explanation that group therapy has been found to provide more stimulus and support than individual treatments.

Group therapy

The 'pelvic floor group' meets once a week for about 20 minutes. Very little equipment is required, any moderate-sized room is suitable.

EXERCISES
Pelvic floor contractions are practised in all the variations of lying, sitting and standing, making the positions relate to the patient's daily life. To prevent fatigue of the pelvic floor muscles, strengthening and mobilizing exercises for the abdominal and back muscles are interspersed. Posture correction is also taught.

As the pelvic floor muscles increase in strength the contractions can be made more difficult to sustain by practising them while skipping, running and jumping. Coughing, sneezing and lifting with the pelvic floor contracted must also be taught. Duplicated reminder lists of exercises will aid the patient's memory as great emphasis is laid on home practice. The overweight patients are weighed each week and their weight is recorded.

Faradism

The author does not use vaginal faradism as part of the programme. If, however, a patient has such gross weakness of her pelvic floor muscles that she can get no sensation of muscular contraction, then vaginal faradism may be used as a sensory stimulus for about six treatments.

METHOD
Individual vaginal electrodes can be made for each patient. A 5 inch (12·5 cm) length of malleable zinc is rolled round a pencil to give it shape. When the pencil is withdrawn all edges are turned in about one

eighth of an inch and the long sides pressed together until they just meet. A lead can then be attached to one end either through a hole in the electrode or a metal clip, to make connection to the faradic source.

With the patient in crook lying a large (6 × 9 inch or 15 × 23 cm) indifferent electrode and wet lint pad is placed under the sacrum. The patient can insert the vaginal electrode herself. If unwilling to do so the therapist will find it easy if she remembers that the vagina angles downwards and backwards in crook lying.

The intensity should be increased until the patient is feeling a strong contraction of her pelvic floor muscles, within the limits of comfort. She should be encouraged to try to contract the muscles actively with the surges a few times in each treatment.

FARADISM UNDER GENERAL ANAESTHESIA
Some authorities have used several maximal faradic stimuli to the perineal body of an anaesthetized patient, and claim this aids the strengthening of the pelvic floor muscles.

SHORT WAVE DIATHERMY

The resolution of some gynaecological conditions can be accelerated by the application of deep heat.

The shortwave diathermic current is of high frequency and alternating, and does not stimulate motor or sensory nerves. It is ideal for heating tissues as deeply placed in the pelvis as the female reproductive organs.

Physiological effects

Shortwave diathermy produces heat in the tissues; the resulting rise in temperature accelerates metabolism and causes an increased blood flow to the area.

Uses

The increased blood flow through the area together with increased flow of oxygen and nutrients and the removal of waste products make the resolution of inflammation the main use of shortwave diathermy in gynaecological conditions. Pain produced by an inflammatory process will also be relieved as the inflammation resolves.

Method

The two most useful methods of arranging the electrodes are crossfire and contraplanar.

CROSSFIRE

The tissues in the pelvis are very vascular and therefore have a very high dielectric constant. The cross-sectional area of the pelvis is larger than that of the electrodes. These two facts combine to make the superficial tissues receive more heat than the deep ones.

To prevent this overheating of the superficial tissues, the field can be passed through the pelvis in two directions. This involves moving the electrodes to a position at right angles to their previous position halfway through the treatment.

In this way half the treatment could be given antero-posteriorly through the pelvis with the patient in the lying position, and the second half with the patient in the side-lying position with legs curled up and the electrodes over the pelvic outlet and the lumbo-sacral area of the spine.

To limit the spreading of the field and encourage deep heating the electrodes should be widely spaced from each other, and air (which has a low dielectric constant) used as a spacer between skin and electrode where possible (Scott, 1969).

CONTRAPLANAR

In conditions which produce vaginal discomfort it is useful to have the distribution of the field uneven, and thus get a concentration of heat over the electrode nearer the skin.

The patient sits low in a deck chair (cotton or linen canvas only) with her thighs apart, with a large flat electrode under her perineum, (with a suitable amount of felt spacers or towelling between her and the electrode). The other electrode can be placed over the abdomen making sure that the skin/electrode spacing is greater than in the other electrode.

Alternatively the perineal electrode could be of the condenser type and be placed under the chair close to the canvas. If the abdomen is heavily scarred the directing electrode could be placed behind the lumbo-sacral region.

A course of 12 treatments each lasting 20 minutes is satisfactory. At least two treatments should be given per week.

Precautions especially relevant in the treatment of gynaecological patients by shortwave diathermy

CLOTHING

The patient should remove all her garments from her waist down to her feet. The skin of the abdomen, buttocks and thighs can be adequately inspected for scars or other blemishes.

SKIN SENSATION

Every area that is to be treated should be tested for sensation to heat and cold, paying particular attention to any scarred area which may show altered reactions.

MOISTURE

Great care should be taken to see that the perineum and inner aspects of the thighs are dry, as moisture will cause a concentration of the field. If the patient is obese a dry turkish towel could be placed between her thighs.

INTRA-UTERINE DEVICES

These contraceptive devices have been found to lose their shape when subjected to shortwave diathermy. Metal devices like the 'Copper 7' concentrate the field.

It is the author's opinion that shortwave diathermy is *contra-indicated* for a patient fitted with an intra-uterine device.

MENSTRUATION

It has been the practice not to treat a patient who is menstruating. The author has found it unnecessary to suspend treatment at this time unless the patient has very heavy periods or secondary dysmenorrhoea.

The sanitary protection should be removed before treatment, whether it is pad or tampon, and the perineum thoroughly dried. The patient can sit on a paper towel if she feels she may soil the towelling. A clean pad or tampon can be replaced after treatment.

The presence of pacemakers, hearing aids or items of replacement surgery should be checked for in the usual way.

Conditions treated by shortwave diathermy

PELVIC INFLAMMATORY DISEASE

Details of this condition are given on page 79. Shortwave diathermy is used in the treatment of the chronic phase of this disease.

CHRONIC CATARRHAL ENDOCERVICITIS

Symptoms of this condition are deep tenderness in the transcervical and uterosacral ligaments, dragging backache, dyspareunia and vaginal discharge.

The cervix of the patient is cauterized under a general anaesthetic. If after three to six weeks there is residual tenderness of the ligaments and dyspareunia, shortwave diathermy will aid resolution.

DISCOMFORT IN THE VAGINA OR INTROITUS

This symptom may be found at the postnatal examination. Shortwave diathermy can hasten the patient's return to normal.

INFERTILITY

Shortwave diathermy may assist in certain cases.

Conclusion

The role of the physiotherapist does not only lie in the treatment of the patient's symptoms as mentioned in this chapter.

Prophylaxis must be her aim. Her knowledge of the musculo-skeletal changes of pregnancy, labour and the puerperium must be used to minimize the effects of these processes on women.

Patient care starts during antenatal classes and should include instruction to the pupil midwives and district midwives who have no obstetric physiotherapist working with them.

Constant attention should be given to postnatal exercise schemes to ensure they contain the right exercises and are taught effectively. Patients in the postnatal ward who have a history of stress incontinence should have the ability to contract their pelvic floor muscles checked in the physiotherapy out-patient department after their postnatal examination. Further teaching and checking should continue for three to six months and if problems occur the gynaecologist should be consulted.

It is by this combination of prophylaxis and active treatment that the physiotherapist can contribute so much in the alleviation of some of the problems of modern women of all age-groups.

BIBLIOGRAPHY

Hutch, J. A. *Anatomy and Physiology of the Bladder, Trigone and Urethra.* Butterworth, 1972.

Gynaecological Conditions

Llewellyn-Jones, D. *Fundamentals of Obstetrics and Gynaecology*, Vol. II Gynaecology. Faber & Faber, 1970.

Mehta, M. *Intractable Pain*. W. B. Saunders, 1973.

Scott, P. M. (ed.). *Clayton's Electrotherapy and Actinotherapy*. Bailliere Tindall, 6th ed. 1969.

Wright, Samson. *Applied Physiology* (revised by C. A. Keele and E. Neil). Oxford University Press, 12th ed. 1971.

FURTHER READING

Garrey, M. M., Govan, A. D. T., Hodge, C. H. and Callander, R. *Gynaecology Illustrated*. Churchill Livingstone, 2nd ed. 1974.

Jeffcoate, T. N. A. *Principles of Gynaecology*. Butterworth, 4th ed. 1975.

Llewellyn-Jones, D. *Fundamentals of Obstetrics and Gynaecology*, Vol. I Obstetrics. Faber & Faber, 2nd ed. 1977.

Philipp, E. E., Barnes, J. and Newton, M. (eds.). *Scientific Foundations of Obstetrics and Gynaecology*. Heinemann, 1970.

CHAPTER 4

Cranial Surgery

by M. C. BALFOUR, MCSP

INTRODUCTION

By means of extensive research more has become known of the central nervous system, although much remains to be discovered. Increasing knowledge of brain areas, pathways, spinal cord tracts and function has opened up new fields in surgical neurology. Improved equipment, techniques, anaesthetics, drugs and antibiotics contribute to reduce the operating time and minimize postoperative complications.

Early diagnosis and admission to a neurosurgical unit is essential to ensure maximum benefit as delay may cause irreparable damage with resultant risk of permanent disability.

It must be remembered that arising from brain lesions, motor and sensory defects may be accompanied by other defects which have a direct bearing on the capabilities of the patient, such as defects in sight, hearing, intellect and speech. Spinal lesions may also be accompanied by some degree of psychological disturbance which requires full understanding and suitable management.

Teamwork is essential in the overall aim to rehabilitate the patient for normal living. The team includes surgeons, nursing staff, physiotherapists, occupational therapists, speech therapists, psychologists and social workers. Interchange of knowledge between members of the team allows a full understanding of the particular problems of each patient. Encouragement, patience and perseverance are of paramount importance during the rehabilitation period, which can be said to begin immediately the patient enters hospital.

Speech therapist

A wide range of speech disorders arise from lesions in the brain and can have a psychological as well as a neurological basis. The following are some of the disorders found:

complete loss of speech;

difficulty in finding the correct word;

understanding what is said but unable to reply;

inco-ordination of speech existing with cerebellar lesions;

voice volume loss and accelerated speech, found with parkinsonism.

A patient with a speech disorder can become very distressed and frustrated, thus guidance from the speech therapist on how to deal with the problem is very important. Information regarding speech recovery is essential to the occupational therapist and physiotherapist. The speech therapist is helped by reports from other departments on how much the patient attempts to speak and how well he makes himself understood. It is important to the patient that he can communicate with people, thus some time should be devoted to speaking to him and to giving him the opportunity and time to reply.

Certain types of speech disorders affect the patient's ability to co-operate with the various therapists. A patient may be unable to understand the spoken word but may understand and respond to written commands. A demonstration by the therapist may be necessary if the patient cannot comprehend the spoken or written word. Great patience is thus required by all members of the rehabilitation team in order to gain full co-operation from the patient.

Psychologist

Information and advice from the psychologist can be invaluable as he plays an important part in assessing the patient's mental state, which is not always easy to do in general conversation. A large range of psychological disturbances is associated with brain lesions and requires to be understood in order to be dealt with successfully and to make allowances for the patient.

In lesions of the dominant cerebral hemisphere (left side in a right-handed person) various types and degrees of loss of motor skills can exist with retention of adequate voluntary power and comprehension. They present as clumsiness or odd errors, which may improve with retraining. In right cerebral hemisphere lesions, 'body scheme' and visual perceptual disorders can exist, leading to odd behaviour such as difficulty with dressing and finding the way about. Patience and persistence in retraining usually meet with improvement unless the lesion is a progressive one.

A general disturbance of cerebral function has a general effect on behaviour, appearing as poor intellect, memory, concentration and grasp of the situation. Associated with these disorders may be a loss of normal control of emotional reactions. This includes undue tendencies to distress and irritability, often alternating with periods of excessive cheerfulness. To gain the patient's co-operation for physiotherapy treatment, firm, tactful management is essential.

Occupational therapist

The work of the occupational therapist is closely linked with that of the physiotherapist. The patient's programme of treatment is such that the retraining of motor and sensory defects along functional lines is shared by both departments. The occupational therapist may require information as to the return and degree of voluntary power to enable her to select an appropriate activity. In turn the physiotherapist is informed of any particular difficulty the patient experiences when attempting these activities, so that she can then concentrate on the re-education of the specific defects.

When a neglect phenomenon is the main feature, bimanual tasks are given to encourage the use of the neglected limb. These tasks are also given when a homonymous hemianopia is present, so encouraging the patient to compensate for loss of visual field by head movements. Loss of sensation in the hand is re-educated by teaching the patient to appreciate objects of different sizes, weights and textures. Writing difficulties are associated with certain brain lesions, notably parkinsonism, the tendency being for the writing to decrease in size. Some speech disorders are accompanied by loss of the ability to write. The physical re-education of writing deficiencies is undertaken by the occupational therapist.

Remedial sports such as skittles, darts, table tennis and archery are useful for the re-education of balance and co-ordination. The patient with a spinal lesion derives particular benefit from archery which strengthens the shoulder girdle muscles and improves balance, and table tennis, which aids balance and co-ordination.

To regain the patient's independence, feeding and dressing are encouraged and gadgets provided when necessary. Kitchen facilities are provided to enable the housewife to practise her culinary skills and adjust to her disability. The need for modifications or the use of certain gadgets in her own kitchen may become apparent. A home visit by the occupational therapist and the physiotherapist to advise as to modifications in all parts of the home is important. Heavy workshop activities which include woodwork are provided for male patients.

Work assessments are carried out as a guide to the type of employment the patient is suited for when his rehabilitation programme is complete.

Social worker

Resettlement problems are dealt with by the social worker working, as do other members of the medical and rehabilitation staff, in close collaboration with the consultant in charge of the patient, who directs investigations and treatment.

The patient who has residual physical and mental defects may be unable to return to his former employment. It may be possible for the social worker to arrange with the local authority for which she works for the provision of certain modifications in the home, such as ramps, rails at strategic places in bathrooms, banister rails, etc., which have been recommended by the physiotherapist. In certain cases it may even be possible to have the patient and his family rehoused.

A patient less severely handicapped may require help to find a suitable retraining scheme for employment within his capabilities. The social worker may help to gain the co-operation of his current employer to re-employ the patient in a job suitable to his capabilities. Financial difficulties can also arise and the social worker may be able to help and advise. Whenever it is possible the patient resumes some form of employment, thus helping him to regain confidence in himself and in his ability to live independently, or relatively so.

During the course of physiotherapy treatment the patient may confide his worries and difficulties or give the impression of being worried and depressed. The physiotherapist should then advise him to see the social worker. There are various occasions when a report on the patient's progress and capabilities in occupational therapy and physiotherapy are useful to the social worker when making appropriate arrangements for employment and housing. It is often in co-operation with the social worker that an optimum discharge date can be decided upon.

When a patient has derived maximum benefit from his physiotherapy treatment and finds it difficult to break this contact, usually due to feelings of insecurity or even loneliness, the social worker may be able to suggest alternative interests such as clubs for the disabled and other organizations interested in the welfare of the disabled.

ANATOMY AND PHYSIOLOGY

For the purpose of description, the brain may be divided into cerebrum, midbrain, pons, medulla oblongata and the cerebellum, which lies behind the two last-named. It must be remembered that the entire mechanism is highly complex, no one part works as a separate entity, and the response of the brain is a result of the integrated action of its various systems.

The following is a brief guide to the effect of a lesion at various levels throughout the brain.

Cerebrum (see Figs. 4/1 and 4/2, 6 below and p. 108)

The cerebrum is the largest part of the brain, and consists of two hemispheres connected by bundles of nerve fibres, the corpus callosum.

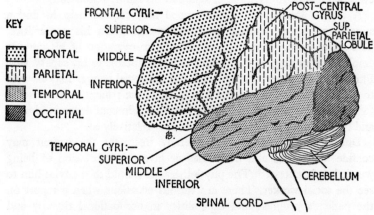

Fig. 4/1 The brain seen from the side.

The surface of each hemisphere covered by layers of cells constitutes the cerebral cortex. This represents the highest centre of function and can be roughly mapped into areas, each concerned with a specific function. To facilitate reference each hemisphere is divided into four lobes, namely frontal, temporal, parietal and occipital. The right hemisphere controls the left side of the body, and the left hemisphere controls the right side of the body and usually controls speech function.

FRONTAL LOBE (see Figs. 4/1 and 4/3)

Area	Function	Effect of a lesion
(A) Motor area (which gives rise to the cerebro-spinal tracts)	Controls voluntary movement of the opposite half of the body which is represented on the cortex in an upside down position	Flaccid paralysis. A lesion between the hemispheres produces paraplegia
(B) Pre-motor area	Localization of motor function	*Spastic paralysis. Psychological changes
(C)	Controls movements of the eyes	The eyes turn to the side of the lesion and cannot be moved to the opposite side
(D)	Motor control of larynx, tongue, and lips to enable movements of articulation	Inability to articulate
(E) 'Silent area'	Believed to control abstract thinking, foresight, mature judgement, tactfulness	Lack of a sense of responsibility in personal affairs

*The effects of a lesion in the pre-motor area vary with the rate of onset; a lesion which occurs suddenly, such as a head injury or a haemorrhage, will result in a flaccid paralysis initially, spasm gradually developing over a variable period of time. A lesion which has a slow mode of onset, such as a slowly growing neoplasm, will produce spasm in the early stages.

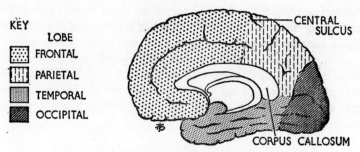

Fig. 4/2 Sagittal section of the brain.

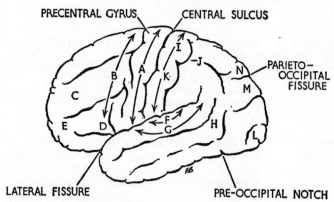

Fig. 4/3 Diagram showing some cortical areas of the brain.

TEMPORAL LOBE (see Figs. 4/1 and 4/3)

Area	Function	Effect of a lesion
(F and G)	Hearing and associ-ation of sound	Inability to localize the direction of sound
(H) Auditory speech area	Understanding of the spoken word	Inability to understand what is said

Other areas on the medial aspect of the temporal lobe are associated with the sense of smell and taste. The optic radiations sweep through the temporal lobe to reach the occipital lobe and these may also be damaged by a lesion of the temporal lobe giving rise to a homonymous hemianopia. (See diagram on Visual Pathways, Fig. 4/6.)

PARIETAL LOBE (see Figs. 4/1 and 4/3)

Area	Function	Effect of a lesion
(I, J and K)	Sensory receptive areas for light touch, two-point discrimination, joint position sense and pressure	Corresponding sensory loss giving rise to a 'neglect phenomenon'. 'Body image' loss is associated with lesions of the non-dominant hemisphere

Visual defects arising from lesions in the parietal area may be highly complex and the patient unaware of them. Sensory loss gives a severe disability, which is out of proportion to any associated voluntary power loss.

OCCIPITAL LOBE (see Figs. 4/1 and 4/3)

Area	Function	Effect of a lesion
(L)	Receptive area for visual impressions	Loss of vision in some areas of the visual fields. (See diagram on Visual Pathways.)
(M and N)	Recognition and interpretation of visual stimuli	Inability to recognize things visually

BRAINSTEM

All nerve fibres to and from the cerebral cortex converge towards the brainstem forming the corona radiata, and on entering the diencephalon they become the internal capsule (see Fig. 4/4, p. 110). When the cerebral cortex is removed the remainder, or central core, is termed the brainstem. Its components from above downwards are: the diencephalon; the basal ganglia; the mesencephalon or midbrain; the pons; and the medulla oblongata.

The nuclei of the cranial nerves are scattered throughout this area.

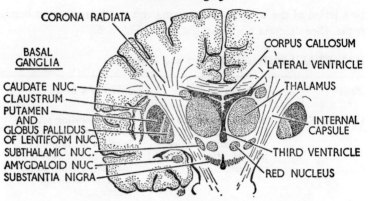

Fig. 4/4 A diagrammatic view of the brain in cross-section.

DIENCEPHALON (see Fig. 4/4.)

Components	Function	Effects of a lesion
(A) Hypothalamus lies in the grey matter near the floor and lower walls of the third ventricle	1. Influences respiration, heart rate and blood pressure 2. Due to its connection with the reticular formation, it influences the conscious level 3. Influences the pituitary gland 4. Influences appetite 5. Has some influence over emotional behaviour 6. Regulation of body temperature 7. Fluid balance	1. Alterations in respiratory and heart rate and blood pressure 2. Pathological sleep 3. Refer to pituitary gland dysfunction 4. Appetite may be increased or decreased 5. Effects on emotional behaviour are very variable 6. Increase in body temperature 7. Diabetes insipidus
(B) The thalamus (refer to Fig. 4/4 for its position). To date over 150 areas have been defined	1. Relays impulses of all types to the cerebral cortex 2. Incomplete but conscious awareness of peripheral sensory stimuli 3. Focusing attention	A posterolateral lesion causes hemiparesis, sensory loss and intractable pain, loss of co-ordination and vasomotor changes. Anterior lesions may cause involuntary movements and impaired sensation. Lesion of the mid-portion may cause mental changes

Basal ganglia

Broadly speaking the basal ganglia include the caudate nucleus, putamen, globus pallidus, amygdala, claustrum, substantia nigra, subthalamic nucleus. The corpus striatum and extrapyramidal motor system refers to the caudate nucleus, putamen and globus pallidus. The subthalamus and substantia nigra are closely related in function to the extrapyramidal motor system.

Lesions of the extrapyramidal system can be divided into two types, hyperkinetic and hypokinetic.

HYPERKINETIC

Examples of hyperkinetic lesions are: chorea, characterized by quick, jerky, purposeless movements; athetosis, which gives slow, writhing movements of the limbs; hemiballismus, causing continual wild, flail-like movements usually confined to one arm.

HYPOKINETIC

This is the parkinsonian syndrome, which will be described later (p. 142).

Midbrain, pons and medulla oblongata

The midbrain, pons and medulla oblongata also act as a funnel for tracts passing from higher levels downwards to the spinal cord and for sensory tracts from the spinal cord passing upwards to higher centres. In view of it being a relatively small area, any lesion can give rise to widespread effects. Involvement of any of the following are likely.

Cerebellar function may be affected due to interference of the efferent and afferent pathways.

Sensation of all types may be affected as the fasciculi gracilis and cuneatus terminate in nuclei in the medulla oblongata. Nerve fibres then arise from these nuclei, cross the mid-line and continue upwards to the thalamus in the medial lemniscus. The spinothalamic tracts which cross in the spinal cord pass directly upwards through the brainstem.

Loss of motor function occurs if the cerebrospinal tracts are damaged. These pass downwards from the internal capsule to decussate at the lower end of the medulla oblongata.

The conscious level can be depressed if there is damage to the reticular formation which is scattered throughout the brainstem.

Vomiting and disturbed respiratory rate can occur with pressure on the vomiting and respiratory centres in the medulla oblongata.

Cranial nerve nuclear lesions may result with characteristic palsies. (see table of cranial nerves, below.)

CRANIAL NERVES (see Fig. 4/5, p. 113)

Cranial nerve	Function	Effect of a lesion
1. Olfactory	Sense of smell	Loss of sense of smell
2. Optic	Vision	Various visual field defects (refer to diagram). Visual acuity affected
3. Oculomotor	Innervates medial, superior, inferior recti and inferior oblique muscle and voluntary fibres of levator palpebrae superioris. Carries autonomic fibres to pupil	Outward deviation of the eye, ptosis, dilation of the pupil
4. Trochlear	Motor supply to the superior oblique eye muscle	Inability to turn the eye downwards and outwards
5. Trigeminal	(a) Motor division to temporalis, masseter, internal and external pterygoid muscles (b) Sensory division: touch, pain and temperature sensation of the face including the cornea on the same side of the body	(a) Deviation of the chin towards the paralysed side when the mouth is open (b) Loss of touch, pain and temperature sensation and of the corneal reflex
6. Abducent	Innervates the external rectus muscle	Internal squint and therefore diplopia
7. Facial	Motor supply to facial muscles on the same side of the body	Paralysis of facial muscles
8. Acoustic	Sensory supply to semicircular canals. Hearing	Vertigo. Nystagmus. Deafness

Cranial nerve	Function	Effect of a lesion
9. Glosso-pharyngeal	Motor to the pharynx. Taste: posterior one-third of the tongue	Loss of gag reflex. Loss of taste in the appropriate area
10. Vagus	Motor to pharynx. Sympathetic and parasympathetic to heart and viscera	Difficulty with swallowing. Regurgitation of food and fluids
11. Accessory	The cranial part of the nerve joins the vagus nerve	
12. Hypoglossal	Motor nerve of the tongue	Paralysis of the side of the tongue corresponding to the lesion, thus it deviates to the paralysed side when protruded

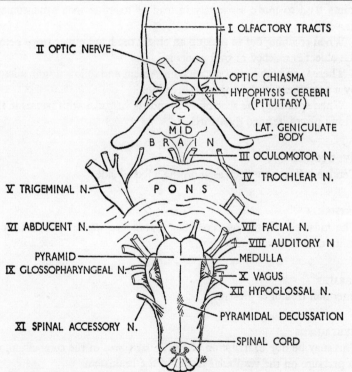

Fig. 4/5 The brain stem and cranial nerves seen from the front.

Cerebellum

The cerebellum lies in the posterior cranial fossa of the skull connected to the pons and medulla oblongata by the cerebellar peduncles. The surface is corrugated and consists of cells forming the cerebellar cortex. It is divided into two cerebellar hemispheres which join near the midline with a narrow middle portion called the vermis.

The cerebellum controls co-ordinate action of muscle groups throughout the body to allow movement to be performed smoothly and accurately. Cerebellar lesions give the following characteristic signs:

ATAXIA

Posture and gait will be disturbed. A unilateral cerebellar lesion causes the patient to overbalance to the side of the lesion.

When performing a movement which involves several joints, the joints tend to move separately instead of together in a synchronized movement.

When reaching out to pick up an object the hand either stops before the object is reached or overshoots it.

There is an inability to stop one movement and follow it immediately by a movement in the opposite direction.

When speaking, the spacing of sounds is irregular with pauses in the wrong places, termed dysarthria.

HYPOTONIA

Tendon reflexes are decreased on the affected side.

ASTHENIA

The muscles affected by cerebellar lesions are weaker and tire more easily than normal muscles.

TREMOR

Intention tremor is present.

NYSTAGMUS

This may be due to irritation of vestibular fibres in the cerebellum, or to pressure on the vestibular nuclei of the brainstem.

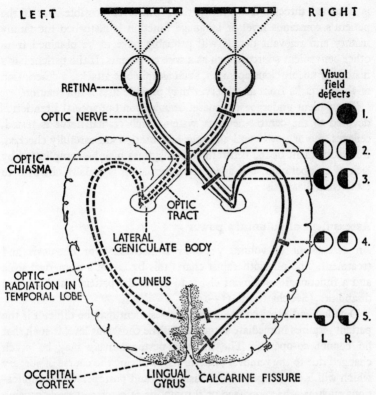

Fig. 4/6 Diagram to show the effects of injury on the visual pathway
1. Shows blindness in one eye.   2. Bitemporal hemianopia.
3. Left homonymous hemianopia.   4 and 5. Quadrantic defects.

EXAMINATIONS AND INVESTIGATIONS

Before surgery can be considered, extensive examinations and investigations may need to be carried out to localize the lesion and decide upon its nature and likely prognosis.

Examinations

A history of the patient's present illness, previous illnesses and any relevant family illness is noted, and social circumstances, occupation, drinking and smoking habits are taken into account. This information is obtained directly from the patient whenever possible, but if the patient's conscious level or language function is disturbed the family history and relevant details will probably have to be obtained from other convenient sources, such as a wife or parents. If the patient has a history of unconscious episodes, such as epileptic attacks, a description of these attacks from an observer may provide useful information.

The patient undergoes a general examination but special attention is devoted to the central nervous system; each cranial nerve is tested, reflexes, motor power and all types of sensation are carefully checked. Full assessment of the central nervous system may be complicated by lack of co-operation, but adequate information is usually obtained to establish a diagnosis.

Assessment of voluntary power

An assessment of voluntary power is necessary for diagnosis and treatment. The physiotherapist charts this by use of a numerical scale and a functional assessment chart, to assess the patient's abilities and disabilities, (See charts, pp. 117–121).

Detailed and precise pre-operative assessment may be difficult if the patient requires immediate surgery, or if the conscious level is such that he cannot co-operate. The findings postoperatively may be much changed due to the removal of brain tissue during the course of surgery which will lead to a permanent disability, and postoperative complications such as a haemorrhage or thrombosis of cerebral vessels causing irreparable damage.

Special investigations

These procedures may be carried out while the patient is having physiotherapy treatment, and this in consequence may need to be modified for a few days.

LUMBAR PUNCTURE

A needle is inserted in the subarachnoid space between the third and fourth lumbar spinous processes; the pressure of the cerebrospinal fluid is determined and a sample of fluid taken for diagnostic purposes. Following lumbar puncture the patient is nursed lying flat in bed for 24 hours, and active physiotherapy can be given in any of the lying positions. A severe headache may develop after a lumbar puncture. This can be relieved by elevating the foot of the bed for several hours during which time no physiotherapy treatment is given.

X-RAY

Plain films of the skull are usually necessary and can be supplemented by special views of various areas. A note is made of any intracranial calcification and possible displacement of a calcified pineal body. General X-ray examination may be indicated and chest X-rays are always taken.

PHYSIOTHERAPY DEPARTMENT
Physical demands of daily living

NAME   AGE   DIAGNOSIS

ADDRESS   DISABILITY

Bed activities	Date	Comments
1. Moving place to place in bed		
2. Rolling to L. and then to R.		
3. Sitting erect in bed		
4. Turn and lie on abdomen		
5. Remove objects from side table		
6. Sitting on edge of bed		

Toilet activities		
1. Manipulating bedpan		
2. Manipulating urinal		
3. Get on and off toilet		
4. Get in and out of bath		

PHYSIOTHERAPY DEPARTMENT
Physical demands of daily living

NAME   AGE   DIAGNOSIS

ADDRESS   DISABILITY

Elevation activities	*Date*	*Comments*
1. Bed to erect		
2. Erect to bed		
3. Wheelchair to standing		
4. Standing to wheelchair		
5. Standing up		
6. Sitting down		
7. Easy chair to erect		
8. Erect to easy chair		
9. Erect to toilet		
10. Toilet to erect		
11. Down to floor		
12. Up from floor		
13. Pick things up from floor		

PHYSIOTHERAPY DEPARTMENT
Physical demands of daily living

NAME	AGE	DIAGNOSIS
ADDRESS	DISABILITY	

Walking activities	*Date*	*Comments*

1. Standing
2. Walking forward
3. Walking backward
4. Running
5. Opening and closing door
   erect position

Gait

1. Four point alternate
2. Swing to
3. Swing through
4. Two point alternate

Climbing activities

1. Up ramp
2. Steps: Handrail
   No handrail
3. Kerbs
4. Bus step

OCCUPATIONAL THERAPY DEPARTMENT
Assessment form 1

NAME   R/L HANDED

Daily living activities	*Pre-operative date*	*Postoperative date*
EATING		
Eat with spoon		
Eat with knife and fork		
Able to cut meat		
Able to butter bread		
Able to drink from feeder/cup/ glass		
WASHING		
Turn water taps		
Wash and dry hands		
Wash and dry face and neck		
Bath self		
Dry self		
Clean teeth, dentures		
Shave/use cosmetics		
Brush/comb hair		
DRESSING		
Underclothes		
Shirt/blouse		
Trousers/skirt		
Jacket/overcoat		
Socks/stockings		
Suspenders		
Shoes/shoe laces		
Tie		
Fastening: buttons/hooks/zips		

OCCUPATIONAL THERAPY DEPARTMENT
Assessment form 2

NAME   R/L HANDED

Manual dexterity	*Pre-operative date*		*Postoperative date*	
	Right handed	*Left handed*	*Right handed*	*Left handed*
Dexterity board, replace 12/24 pegs				
Match from box and strike it				
Thread 12 washers on rod				
Screw lid off and on jar				
Open and close safety pin				
Pick 12 pins up and stick in cushion				
Fold and envelope letter				
Open letter				
Manage book and turn pages				
Turn newspaper inside out				
Take 3 coins from purse/pocket				
Turn door handle, knob, lever				
Insert door key and turn lock				
Ability to use scissors				

ECHO-ENCEPHALOGRAPHY

By means of ultrasonic waves echoes from mid-line structures can be obtained and mass lesions causing displacements can be detected easily and safely and may serve to indicate the need for further appropriate investigations.

LUMBAR AIR ENCEPHALOGRAPHY

Small quantities of air are injected after lumbar puncture with the patient seated erect. Films are taken with the patient successively erect, supine and prone. The whole ventricular system, the basal cisterns and the subarachnoid spaces are displayed showing any displacements or deformities, thus accurately indicating the site of any lesions. Improved X-ray tubes and television screening have allowed better detail to be produced and the use of tomography allows a more detailed study. Tomography is more extensively practised with particular reference to the petrous bones. Nursing care and physiotherapy treatment are the same as following lumbar puncture.

VENTRICULOGRAPHY
A burr hole is drilled in the skull allowing insertion of a needle into a lateral ventricle. Myodil, a radio-opaque solution, or air, is then introduced and manoeuvred into the third and fourth ventricles. This procedure is often used to demonstrate lesions in the posterior fossa, and is a routine measure during stereotaxic surgery, when it is used to outline appropriate cerebral landmarks. This allows accurate measurements to be made, which are necessary for the introduction of electrodes into chosen positions. Nursing care and physiotherapy treatment are as previously described.

CEREBRAL ANGIOGRAPHY
This is an extremely important procedure, which is usually carried out under a general anaesthetic. Injections of radio-opaque solutions into the carotid or vertebral arteries are followed by taking films of the arterial, capillary and venous phases of the circulation. Displacement of the blood vessels shows the site of intracranial masses such as clots, tumours, abscesses or cysts. In a proportion of tumour cases, the circulation of the tumour itself may also be seen and may give an accurate assessment of its pathological type.

Angiography is of great value in cerebro-vascular disease. The site of arterial stenosis or occlusion is easily seen. In spontaneous intracranial haemorrhage the site of an aneurysm or arteriovenous anomaly can only be determined by angiography. Postoperative angiography is a useful means of checking the efficiency of surgical treatment of aneurysms and anomalies.

Indirect methods of angiography are now more frequently used. A catheter is inserted into the femoral or axillary artery and its tip passed into the aortic arch. Large quantities of contrast medium injected under pressure allow the display of all major cerebral arteries.

Following angiography the patient is nursed flat for 24 hours, then allowed to sit up and get out of bed if no headache is present. Physio-therapy treatment consists of breathing exercises and maintenance exercises. If the femoral or axillary artery has been used, care must be taken to ensure that the patient maintains full range of hip or shoulder joint movement.

THERMOGRAPHY

This has only a very limited use in cerebral cases as it only gives information about surface circulation, which is not often directly related to cerebral circulation except in a few cases of obstructive vascular disease.

RADIO-ISOTOPE SCANNING

This is a routine examination for all suspected intracranial tumour cases. There is approximately an 85% success rate. Introduction of isotopes into the cerebrospinal fluid is now used for the study of obstructions to the C.S.F. circulation and helps to distinguish between cerebral atrophy and hydrocephalus with gross increase of intracranial pressure.

MONITORING INTRACRANIAL PRESSURE

A monitoring device can be used to measure intracranial pressure over a period of approximately 48 hours. The information gained allows fuller assessment of the patient's condition and his further management. (This means of measuring intracranial pressure over a period of time has been extremely useful in the management of certain head injury patients whose condition has remained static for no apparent reason. The monitoring can show up huge variations in pressure over a long period, which could go undetected with random measurements, and can indicate the need for a 'shunt' to reduce intracranial pressure, with a resultant improvement in the patient's condition.)

Electro-encephalography

The electro-encephalograph amplifies and records the electrical activity of the brain, but it can only give a measure of the extent of the disorder of brain function. No abnormal E.E.G. pattern is specific to the disease which produces it, thus interpretation of records requires an appreciation of the clinical problems involved and close liaison between the interpreter and the clinician. An E.E.G. can be recorded within 45 minutes, with no danger or discomfort to the patient.

Many problems exist which E.E.G. cannot at present solve; however there are groups of cases in which it can be of real value. It must be appreciated that E.E.G. does not give a definitive diagnosis, but merely provides information which is of help in the final clinical evaluation of any particular case. Some of the useful applications to surgical neurology are:

Outpatients can be screened, particularly those suffering from headaches and bizarre psychiatric symptoms. An unsuspected organic lesion in a silent area of the brain may be divulged which can then be dealt with surgically.

An E.E.G. can be used to help distinguish between cerebral tumours and cerebrovascular accidents. In the former the E.E.G. abnormality is usually out of proportion to the clinical signs, the reverse being the case in cerebrovascular accidents.

It can also provide positive evidence of a subdural haematoma.

An E.E.G. can help to select those patients with intractable epilepsy who may be helped by surgical excision of a part of the brain. Such patients are those with essentially normal E.E.G.s, who show a defined focus of abnormality in an area of the brain which it is possible to remove surgically.

Electrocorticography, the recording from the exposed brain at operation, may help particularly in cases of epilepsy, to decide which areas are abnormal and responsible for the patient's fits.

GENERAL SIGNS AND SYMPTOMS OF CEREBRAL LESIONS

Raised intracranial pressure

Intracranial pressure depends on the volume of the skull contents. In a child under the age of 18 months, any slow increase in volume will result in an increase in the size of the head. In individuals over the age of 18 months there is no increase in the size of the head, thus the effects of raised intracranial pressure will produce a disturbance of cerebral function more rapidly. Increased volume may be caused by a space-occupying lesion, such as a tumour or abscess, a blockage in the cerebrospinal fluid pathways or by haemorrhage from an aneurysm.

Symptoms of raised intracranial pressure

With raised intracranial pressure the soft-walled veins become compressed, giving rise to oedema and subsequent lack of oxygen to the brain tissue, the symptoms varying with the degree of raised pressure. The most common factors arising are as follows:

HEADACHE
This is probably due to abnormal tensions in the cerebral blood vessels. In the early stages this may be paroxysmal, occurring during the night and early morning. With continued increase in pressure it becomes continuous and is intensified by exertion, coughing and stooping. The headache usually becomes worse when the patient is lying down and is relieved when sitting up.

PAPILLOEDEMA
This is oedema of the optic discs which can cause enlargement of the blind spot and subsequent deterioration of visual acuity and complete blindness.

VOMITING
This occurs when the headache is most severe and tends to be projectile in nature.

PULSE AND BLOOD PRESSURE
Acute and sub-acute rises in pressure cause a slowing of the pulse rate, but if pressure continues to rise the pulse rate becomes very rapid. A rapid increase in intracranial pressure causes a rise in the blood pressure, but a chronic rise does not affect it, and in some lesions below the tentorium cerebelli the blood pressure is below normal.

RESPIRATORY RATE
This is not affected by a slow rise in pressure but a sufficiently rapid increase in pressure, which produces a loss of consciousness, usually results in slow deep respirations. This may change after a period and become irregular, of the Cheyne-Stokes type.

MENTAL SYMPTOMS
These can vary from confusion and disorientation to complete loss of consciousness.

EPILEPTIC CONVULSIONS

Generalized fits may occur but it is not clear whether these are caused by the raised intracranial pressure or by the actual lesion itself.

Eye symptoms

It is essential to realize that eye symptoms are often present with a brain lesion and they can directly affect a patient's capabilities during his rehabilitation. Among those most commonly found are:

Damage to the optic nerve, optic chiasma or optic tracts will cause field defects. (See Fig. 4/6.)

Damage to the third cranial nerve can cause a ptosis, an inability to open the eye.

Nystagmus. This is frequently present in cerebellar or brainstem lesions and is an involuntary jerky movement of the eyes.

Diplopia or double vision. This is present if there is any imbalance of the eye muscles and can be overcome by covering alternate eyes on alternate days until the imbalance adjusts itself.

Ear symptoms

Deafness may be caused by tumours of the eighth cranial nerve such as acoustic neurinomas; these tumours may give rise to vertigo.

Speech disorders

These have already been briefly mentioned in relation to the role of the speech therapist (p. 103). They are mainly associated with lesions of the temporal lobe on the dominant side.

The level of consciousness

Numerous factors can be responsible for alteration in the level of consciousness. Several of the factors are as follows:

certain types of trauma producing a craniocerebral injury;

space-occupying masses causing increased intracranial pressure;

operational trauma;

postoperative complications such as oedema or haemorrhage.

The following are a guide to assessing the patient's conscious level:

(*i*) The patient is fully conscious.

(*ii*) The patient is disorientated with respect to time and space but can answer questions.

(*iii*) The patient can obey commands but cannot answer.

(*iv*) The patient responds to painful stimuli but not to the spoken word.

(*v*) The patient is completely unresponsive.

To assess accurately the patient's conscious level any disturbance of hearing, vision and speech function must always be taken into account, and suitable measures taken to ensure the patient is given every opportunity to understand what is expected of him.

CRANIAL SURGERY

Conditions which may be improved with surgery are as follows:

Cerebral trauma, i.e. craniocerebral (head) injuries (see Chapter VII, *Neurology for Physiotherapists*).

Cerebrovascular disease. This can be divided into haemorrhagic lesions, such as intracranial aneurysms and intracranial angiomatous malformations (arteriovenous anomalies), and ischaemic lesions such as carotid artery stenosis.

Cerebral infections, e.g. intracranial abscesses.

Neoplastic lesions, such as cerebral tumours, cerebellar tumours and acoustic neurinomas.

Dyskinesias, e.g. parkinsonism.

Hydrocephalus.

Epilepsy.

Intractable pain.

The preparation of a patient for a cranial operation is extremely important. In the majority of operations involving the brain, the hair must be totally removed and the scalp carefully prepared. The female patient may require reassurance if she becomes distressed at the prospect. Most operations are performed under general anaesthetic and take a considerable period of time to complete. During the course of surgery a bone flap may be turned back, but this is usually replaced at the end of the operation.

Postoperative treatment

On return from theatre the patient will have a pressure bandage on the head to control swelling; this may be extended to include the eye on the side corresponding to the operational site, for the same purpose. Eyes are very vulnerable to swelling and do so as a result of operational trauma. The position of the patient on the operating table may also be a contributory factor, hence for the first two or three postoperative days the patient may be unable to open either eye. Any intravenous infusion set up in theatre may be continued for the first postoperative day.

Care must be taken to restrain a restless, confused patient, as he may attempt to remove head dressings, which will allow easy access of infection and meningitis may result. Padding and bandages on the hands, which may need to be tied down, reduce this danger. Cot sides should be attached to the bed in the early postoperative phase. It is important to replace hand bandages and cot sides after any treatment.

BONE FLAP

This may be removed if the brain is very swollen during operation, or if the skull is splintered as a result of a head injury. Replacement of this flap is advisable once oedema has subsided, as the patient tends to suffer from headache, dizziness when stooping and is afraid of damage from a bump to the area. Following head injury the bone may be so badly damaged it has to be discarded, and the defect is then filled with plastic material.

When bone has been removed the patient is not nursed on the affected side until he shows signs of recovery of his conscious level. The young active male who is once more ambulant may be provided with a protective metal plate inside a cap, or a crash helmet to prevent further trauma, until the defect is repaired.

VENTRICULAR DRAINAGE

The patient may return from theatre with ventricular drainage if there are signs of blocked cerebrospinal fluid pathways at operation. A catheter is introduced into a lateral ventricle by means of a burr hole in the skull and the cerebrospinal fluid drained into a flask; the height of the flask is dependent upon the pressure of the cerebrospinal fluid. Care should be taken when treating the patient to ensure that the level of the head is not altered in relation to the flask as this alters the drainage pressure.

If the doctor's permission has been given for postural drainage, the height of the flask must be adjusted as the bed is tipped and readjusted on its return to the horizontal, this being done under medical supervision.

Cranial Surgery

LUMBAR DRAINAGE

This may be set up several days postoperatively if there are signs of continued raised intracranial pressure. The needle is placed as for a lumbar puncture and rubber tubing connects it to a drainage flask, the height of which is dependent upon the cerebrospinal fluid pressure. If the drainage is to be continuous the patient is nursed in side lying, well supported by pillows. Turning is done by lifting the patient from side to front, to his other side.

During the first few postoperative days intensive nursing care is required, the patient's condition being carefully observed and charted. Deterioration can occur very rapidly due to postoperative complications, thus any change must be reported immediately as it can be a matter of life and death.

Complications

Apart from the complications arising from brain damage the following may also arise:

Cerebrospinal fluid may leak following the original operation, which may require further surgical repair.

Postoperative oedema, thrombosis or haemorrhage from cerebral blood vessels, occurs in a small number of patients.

Thrombosis may occur elsewhere and pulmonary embolus.

Epilepsy may develop after a variable period of time.

Respiratory complications are fairly common.

Respiratory complications

Postoperative oedema can cause pressure on the respiratory centre and the vagus nerves in the medulla oblongata, causing alteration in the respiratory rate and loss of the cough reflex. The ability to swallow may also be lost, thus there is a constant danger of aspiration of mucus and vomit. Until the ability to swallow returns the patient is artificially fed by means of a Ryle's tube passed down the nose into the stomach to prevent aspiration of food or fluids.

Dealing with chest complications following cranial surgery is made more difficult by postural drainage being contra-indicated immediately after operation, as it will cause an increase in intracranial pressure. Changes in blood pressure may also govern the position in which the patient must remain and it is imperative to check the patient's chart.

If the patient has a raised blood pressure, his head may be elevated about 30 degrees in an attempt to control this, and he must remain in this position. Permission to begin postural drainage should therefore be obtained from the surgeon.

When the conscious level is disturbed one must constantly try to gain the patient's co-operation. Deep breathing must be encouraged and use of pressure on the sides of the chest when the patient breathes out is helpful. Clear orders to cough should be given accompanied by pressure of the hands on the sides of the chest as the patient breathes out. A demonstration of a cough by the physiotherapist can be helpful.

SUCTION

When a patient's conscious level is depressed, or he is conscious but incapable of coughing, suction may be necessary to remove secretions. Shaking, clapping and rib-springing help to loosen secretions. A patient who requires suction is most successfully treated by two people, either a physiotherapist and a nurse or two physiotherapists, one using the suction apparatus while the other assists the patient with breathing and attempts to cough.

TRACHEOSTOMY

This may be necessary if the patient has carbon dioxide retention due to respiratory insufficiency, or a clear airway cannot be maintained by use of a mouth airway and suction. Tracheostomy is also required to deal with the hypersecretions associated with midbrain damage following a head injury.

The removal of secretions from a patient with a tracheostomy should be regarded as an aseptic technique, the physiotherapist masked and gowned and the hands well scrubbed before touching the suction catheters.

Chest work with a patient who has respiratory complications can be very time-consuming and it may take almost constant attention throughout the day, but it is well worth the time and effort. An 'on call' system for physiotherapists is necessary when a patient has respiratory complications, which allows the patient to have chest care at any time throughout the 24-hour period.

General physiotherapy treatment

The aims are to prevent chest complications, to maintain circulation, and to make any pertinent assessment of the patient.

METHODS

The patient must be told that the anaesthetic may act as an irritant, causing the production of excess chest secretions. Breathing exercises are taught and he is told to practise them hourly before operation and as soon as he recovers from the anaesthetic. A check must be made on the patient's ability to cough. It should be tactfully suggested that smoking is cut down or stopped for a few days.

The patient must be told to keep his legs moving after operation to maintain his circulation. Maintenance exercises are then taught which he may practise before operation and at hourly intervals postoperatively. This minimizes the danger of deep venous thrombosis. Passive movements are substituted when the patient has a loss of voluntary power.

Assessment of voluntary power loss, degree of ataxia, and type of gait is carried out where the patient's condition allows.

These general principles apply to all conditions in this chapter and the following one; they are modified and adapted to the patient's specific needs. The physiotherapy treatment following each of the conditions listed will therefore be confined to specific points.

INTRACRANIAL ANEURYSMS

Intracranial aneurysms are balloon-like dilatations occurring at the bifurcation of vessels in the circulus arteriosus. The precipitating cause is thought to be a defect in the wall of the blood vessel of congenital origin. Aneurysms are also associated with arteriosclerosis and hypertension. The size varies from a pea to a plum and multiple aneurysms may be present. Age-groups most affected are individuals between 30 and 50 years old.

Rupture of an aneurysm is the most common cause of spontaneous subarachnoid haemorrhage. Signs and symptoms from such a haemorrhage naturally depend on the severity and site of the bleeding. A minor leak from an aneurysm gives sudden severe neck pain, the pain then radiates up over the head and settles to a generalized headache and stiffness of the neck. Severe haemorrhage will cause increased intracranial pressure and loss of consciousness with various neurological deficiencies, depending on the degree of damage from the haemorrhage.

INVESTIGATIONS

The investigations to establish the diagnosis are: *lumbar puncture*, to establish the presence of blood in the cerebrospinal fluid, and *angiography*, to determine the exact site of the aneurysm.

Surgical treatment

Unless an attempt is made surgically to deal with the aneurysm there is a constant danger of further haemorrhage which can be fatal.

To obtain a satisfactory result, operative procedure is undertaken only if the patient is conscious and showing improvement from any neurological deficits arising from the initial bleeding. All procedures are directed towards occluding the aneurysm by one of the following methods: by use of clips; by a clip and wrapping the aneurysm in muslin gauze or muscle; or by clipping the feeding vessel intracranially to reduce the force of blood entering the aneurysm.

Physiotherapy treatment

The patient is taught breathing exercises and how to cough. If the level of consciousness is depressed suction may be necessary to remove secretions.

Passive movements may be given if there are motor deficiencies.

All muscles which are active will be strengthened and maintained and facilitation techniques used to re-educate weak muscles.

If no complications occur as a result of operation the patient will be allowed to get out of bed on about the fifth day. Prior to getting up, the head of the bed is slowly elevated until the patient can tolerate sitting up.

Balance re-education begins with the patient sitting on the edge of the bed with his feet supported. His blood pressure may require checking. A significant rise or fall will necessitate his return to bed, otherwise he can progress to balance in standing, a short walk, then return to bed.

Walking re-education will require minimum attention if no motor deficiencies were present after surgery. If a hemiparesis does exist re-education will be necessary.

PROGRESSION OF TREATMENT

The patient is allowed up for progressively longer periods and gradually takes over his own personal care such as bathing, dressing and going to the toilet.

His rehabilitation programme in both physiotherapy and occupational therapy departments is increased until he can cope with a full programme without undue fatigue, and demonstrate his ability to live independently.

Complications

Further bleeding from the aneurysm may occur while the surgeon is attempting to obliterate it. This may lead to further damage to the brain with a resultant increase in neurological defects.

Traction upon blood vessels in the field of surgery can cause ischaemia of the brain area they supply, which may be severe enough to give rise to defects.

Oedema and thrombosis may follow surgery, and may be severe enough to disturb the conscious level. These postoperative complications manifest themselves 48 hours after surgery and can completely alter the patient's prognosis.

The rehabilitation of a patient suffering from these complications may be either as for the unconscious patient, or as for the patient with hemiplegia or hemiparesis (see *Neurology for Physiotherapists*, Chapters VII and XIII respectively).

LIGATION OF THE COMMON CAROTID ARTERY

This is carried out when certain aneurysms are difficult to approach by a direct method and only if the patient is neurologically intact, or nearly so. If there is an adequate cross-circulation in the brain, the vessel is ligated in the neck under local anaesthetic. If cross-circulation is not adequate a clamp is put on the vessel and the vessel occluded over a period of 48 hours, then finally ligated.

POSTOPERATIVE TREATMENT
The patient is nursed lying flat on the back with a thin pillow under the head and sandbags at either side to stop head movements. A constant check is kept on the blood pressure, pulse rate, conscious level, motor power and the reaction of the pupils to light, in case the patient's condition shows signs of deterioration.

Forty-eight hours after occlusion of the artery the patient can be gradually elevated in bed. Side lying is allowed on approximately the third day. To minimize the risk of any thrombus formation (at the site of the ligation) breaking off during turning, the patient holds his head in his hands, so effectively reducing neck movement.

The patient is allowed to get out of bed on about the seventh day. Prior to getting up he must be able to tolerate sitting erect in bed. His blood pressure must be checked before he is allowed to sit over the edge of the bed, when he achieves this position and when he returns to bed after being up. Any significant drop in blood pressure necessitates return to bed.

Physiotherapy treatment

The patient must be treated gently, to disturb him as little as possible; maintenance exercises which are practised hourly should be reduced to foot movements and static muscle contractions of the leg, abdominal and back muscles.

When the patient is ready to get up, balance re-education may be required in sitting up, then in standing, followed by walking.

PROGRESSION OF TREATMENT

The patient is allowed first to get up and sit in a chair for increasing periods of time, then to walk increasing distances, and then to go up and down stairs.

All progressions must be gently regulated, warning being given to the patient to change his position slowly as a rapid change causes dizziness; thus he must take his time when getting out of bed, standing up or turning round.

His stay in hospital is usually short and on discharge home he is instructed to continue with the slow, gradual resumption of normal activities.

INTRACRANIAL ANGIOMATOUS MALFORMATIONS (ARTERIOVENOUS ANOMALIES)

These malformations are congenital abnormalities of vascular development and occur on the surface of the brain or within the brain tissue, deriving a blood supply from one or both hemispheres, usually found in the younger age-groups including children. Most of the lesions are arteriovenous malformations. The blood vessels of the malformation show degeneration of their walls, and direct communication between arteries and veins in some areas. If the malformation is small no diversion of blood from the capillary bed occurs, but a large one robs the brain of its blood supply.

Signs and symptoms

These are variable but the following may occur: headaches of a migrainous character; focal epilepsy; subarachnoid haemorrhage; spastic monoparesis or hemiparesis together with a sensory or visual loss.

INVESTIGATIONS
Electro-encephalography may be used for diagnosing the cause of headaches and epilepsy. *Angiography* will serve to display the malformation.

Surgical treatment

A direct intracranial approach is made and the lesion excised (if it lies on the surface). Sometimes very complex lesions may be treated by occlusion of the feeding vessels.

PHYSIOTHERAPY TREATMENT
This follows the same course as previously described for aneurysms (p. 132).

CAROTID ARTERY OCCLUSION

Arteriosclerosis with thrombus formation is the usual cause of common and internal carotid artery occlusion. The site of occlusion is most frequently at the origin of the internal carotid artery, and occlusion may be complete or incomplete.

The disease may be of the ischaemic type, which cuts off the blood supply to the involved cerebral hemisphere. Any blood reaching the hemisphere is dependent upon a collateral circulation from the opposite side.

Alternatively the disease may be of the multiple emboli type which continually shoots off small emboli from the site of the occlusion. Anticoagulants such as Dindevan and heparin are necessary for the management of this type.

Signs and symptoms

A wide variety of symptoms and modes of onset can be produced by carotid artery occlusion.

Hemiplegia. This may be profound and occurs suddenly, with loss of consciousness usually accompanying this type of onset. There may be hemiparesis progressing to hemiplegia. There is transient motor weakness ('stuttering') usually affecting one extremity.

Dysphasia, sensory loss and various *eye symptoms* are associated in some degree with the loss of voluntary power.

Headache behind the eye is often present.

INVESTIGATIONS

By means of *angiography* any occlusion is immediately revealed.

Surgical treatment

In carefully selected cases surgery is of great value. Contra-indications are gross arteriosclerotic involvement of other cerebral vessels, and loss of consciousness with the onset of symptoms, which carries a poor prognosis.

Surgical measures aim to restore the normal blood flow and prevent further progression of the disease.

ENDARTERECTOMY

The arteriosclerotic portion of the artery and any thrombus is removed. If the arteriosclerotic area is too extensive, a bypass arterial graft is done.

Physiotherapy treatment

Immediate measures are required for the re-education of the hemiplegic limbs. Bearing in mind the likely sensory loss and field defects of the eyes, the patient must be constantly reminded of the affected limbs. The position of the affected limbs should be checked regularly to reduce the danger of damage to joints, and circulatory obstruction. Passive movements and facilitation techniques should be used to re-educate the affected muscles and the patient must be able to watch his limbs.

Balance and re-education in sitting aided by use of a mirror can begin when the patient is allowed to get up, approximately between the fifth and seventh day.

Walking re-education is also aided by use of a mirror.

During mat work the patient must first be taught to adjust the position of his affected arm and leg before rolling and similar activities.

When sitting in a chair he must constantly be reminded to check the position of his limbs. When walking unaided he must also be taught constantly to check that his foot is not catching on objects in his path, and that he allows ample clearance going through doorways and when walking near a wall.

INTRACRANIAL ABSCESS

Infection causing an intracranial abscess can reach the brain by:

spreading from a nearby source such as otitis media, mastoiditis or sinusitis;

direct introduction from a stab wound which penetrates the skull;

being blood-borne from another source of infection in the body such as a lung abscess or chronic bronchitis; or

from unknown sources.

The rate of growth of an abscess depends on the organism causing the infection. Many abscesses become encapsulated, allowing the surgeon to drain them more easily or effect a complete removal.

Signs and symptoms

These are very similar to those produced by cerebral tumours, that is headache and vomiting, but abscesses tend to give more intellectual upsets and the onset is more rapid; fever and meningitis also occur.

Surgical treatment

This is by complete removal where possible, or by evacuation of pus from the abscess cavity. A drain is then inserted and antibiotics introduced. A check is kept on the size of the cavity by coating the walls with a radio-opaque solution and X-raying the area at two-day intervals.

POSTOPERATIVE TREATMENT

The patient with an intracranial abscess is strictly barrier-nursed and is not allowed to mix with other patients in the ward until the infection has been effectively controlled.

PHYSIOTHERAPY TREATMENT
The rate of progress will be governed by the patient's general condition. Any voluntary power loss will be re-educated by use of facilitation techniques.

A patient with no complications will be allowed to get up on about the fifth postoperative day and can begin a full rehabilitation programme in the occupational and physiotherapy departments as soon as the surgeon's permission has been given.

INTRACRANIAL TUMOURS

Tumours found in and around the brain can be classified into:

PRIMARY TUMOURS
These are either *malignant* of the glioma type (the malignancy of a tumour is judged upon its rate of growth and its tendency to infiltrate the brain tissue), or *benign,* such as the meningiomas.

SECONDARY TUMOURS
These are blood-borne metastases from primary tumours mainly in the lung and breast.

The rate of growth of a tumour is very variable depending on whether it is malignant or benign. Tumours of the glioma type invade the brain substance making complete removal difficult. Types like the meningioma do not invade the brain, but present problems in view of their size and extreme vascularity.

The location of a tumour is the most important factor irrespective of its pathology, because it may involve the vital centres, thus directly threatening the patient's life, or limiting surgical accessibility.

SIGNS AND SYMPTOMS
Some degree of raised intracranial pressure usually exists. Focal signs develop pointing to the site of the tumour.

SURGICAL TREATMENT
This is undertaken where possible with a view to affecting a complete removal of the tumour. Following an incomplete removal, the tumour

may recur. If the tumour is radio-sensitive a course of deep X-ray therapy will follow surgery to shrink or destroy the remaining tumour cells, so increasing the patient's life expectancy.

Intrinsic tumours in the left temporo-parietal area are not usually removed surgically as severe defects would result, namely dysphasia and hemiplegia. Management may be as follows:

For a cystic type of tumour, the cyst is drained so relieving pressure in the area.

A minute part of the tumour is removed for biopsy, deep X-ray may then follow if the tumour is radio-sensitive, or injections of ethoglucid (Epodyl) which also destroys tumour cells.

Bone can be removed to effect a decompression.

Tumours of the brainstem area are rare, but surgical intervention is often contra-indicated in view of the fatal damage which could result.

PHYSIOTHERAPY TREATMENT

A patient without complications is allowed to get up on about the fifth day.

The patient with a hemiparesis or hemiplegia will be treated as described in *Neurology for Physiotherapists*, Chapters XIII and XIV.

Cerebellar tumours

The majority of cerebellar tumours arise in or near the mid-line and may extend into one or both hemispheres, such as the medulloblastomas and astrocytomas, and are commoner in young people.

SIGNS AND SYMPTOMS

These differ considerably depending on the site of the tumour. The following occur in varying degrees:

Raised intracranial pressure;

Hypotonia;

Ataxia; this is probably most marked when the patient is walking. Ataxia is the result of the inability to stabilize the background activity essential for co-ordinated movement. Repeated movement tends to increase ataxia.

Giddiness;

Nystagmus;

Disturbance of function of some cranial nerves;

Sensory loss may occur but it is the exception, not the rule.

SURGICAL TREATMENT

To excise this type of tumour a Cushing's crossbow incision is used involving the arch of the atlas and a craniectomy of the occipital bone.

POSTOPERATIVE TREATMENT

Due to operative trauma and postoperative oedema, the ninth, tenth and eleventh cranial nerves may be temporarily out of action, causing loss of the cough reflex and inability to swallow.

Nursing care is of importance. The patient must be nursed in side lying to prevent possible aspiration of vomit and mucus, and he is artificially fed by Ryle's tube until he is able to swallow. This further reduces the risk of aspiration of food or fluids.

Physiotherapy treatment

Breathing exercises must be practised by the patient. Suction may be necessary to remove secretions until the cough reflex returns. Even after return of the cough reflex, suction may still be required, as the patient becomes quickly exhausted.

Other aims of treatment are to strengthen the general musculature with particular attention to the neck muscles, and to re-educate balance and co-ordination.

Methods. As the patient's condition improves postoperatively exercises can be given to strengthen the general musculature, particularly the back extensor muscles. Re-education of the neck muscles begins with static contractions on about the seventh day and active exercises when sutures are removed about the tenth day.

Re-education of co-ordination begins in bed. The patient will find it easier to produce a co-ordinate movement against resistance, thus re-education can begin with resisted exercises for the ataxic limbs; and holding a certain position against resistance from varying directions (this is termed stabilizing).

Balance re-education begins when the patient is allowed to get up, usually between the fifth and seventh days. Balance is re-educated in sitting on the edge of the bed by means of the stabilizing technique already described.

PROGRESSION OF TREATMENT

It must be emphasized that a patient with a cerebellar lesion fatigues quickly. He will probably have a history of vomiting for a variable period of time before operation, leading to debility and dehydration. His programme of treatment in the physiotherapy and occupational therapy departments must be carefully graded to guard against exhaustion.

As his condition improves the following progressions will be made:

Mat work. Resisted exercises are more accurately carried out than free exercises, thus mat work begins with resisted activities such as rolling, hip raising. Stabilizing is done in each new position.

Activities are progressed to rolling from side to front to the other side. Sitting up from lying down and moving up and down and from side to side on the mat, using the arms to lift the buttocks off the mat. From prone lying practice in getting to the hands and knees position, sitting over from side to side and practice in crawling in all directions. From the hands and knees attaining the kneeling position, then half kneeling, then standing. Resisted crawling in all directions greatly helps balance and co-ordination.

Walking. Parallel bars and a mirror are of great value in the early stages. Stabilizing in standing and resisted walking, walking forwards, backwards and sideways helps to regain the patient's self-confidence. Resistance against the head helps to steady a grossly ataxic patient.

If a walking aid is necessary to gain the patient's independence, elbow crutches or a reciprocal walking aid are more easily managed by the more ataxic patient. A stick may be adequate to support a less severely handicapped person.

Acoustic neurinoma

This tumour arises from the sheath of the eighth cranial nerve.

SIGNS AND SYMPTOMS

There is tinnitus at first, then deafness as the tumour grows.

Vertigo is present.

A facial nerve lesion is produced as compression of the seventh nerve occurs.

Loss of the corneal reflex, and loss of sensations of pain and temperature occur with compression of the fifth cranial nerve.

Ataxia of the limbs on the side of the tumour occurs with compression of the cerebellar hemisphere and cerebellar peduncles.

SURGICAL TREATMENT

The tumour can be completely excised, which usually results in sacrificing the facial nerve.

POSTOPERATIVE TREATMENT

The patient may have swallowing difficulties and loss of the cough reflex; this requires the same nursing care as for a cerebellar tumour (p. 140). Because of the facial nerve palsy the patient will be unable to close his eye, and an eye-glass will be provided to prevent damage to the cornea, and to prevent infection. The nurse devotes special care to the eye until the patient's condition allows a tarsorrhaphy (this is a suturing together of the upper and lower lid). Vision of the eye is thus reduced, which must be remembered during rehabilitation.

PHYSIOTHERAPY TREATMENT

The patient is given breathing exercises and attempts to cough. Suction may be necessary to remove secretions until the cough reflex has fully recovered. The patient practises his breathing exercises hourly.

The re-education of balance and co-ordination are as previously described for cerebellar ataxia (p. 139). Progress can be more rapid as the patient does not fatigue so quickly.

PARKINSONIAN SYNDROME

This syndrome results from lesions of the corpus striatum. The causes are:

Primary degeneration may occur, mainly between 50 and 60 years of age. This condition is found more frequently in males.

Encephalitis lethargica develops in its chronic stage into parkinsonism, affecting any age-group and both sexes equally.

Cerebral arteriosclerosis can also produce this syndrome, occurring mainly in late middle and old age.

Parkinsonism is a progressive disease, the rate of progress being variable.

Signs and symptoms

These may occur unilaterally or bilaterally.

Tremor. The tremor may occur at rest and be diminished by voluntary muscular effort, or it may be aggravated by action, or it may be a mixture of the two.

One or more limbs may be affected together with the face, eyelids, tongue, jaw and neck. Tremor is increased by tension, excitement and concentration. In company it is always worse and can be a great social nuisance.

Rigidity. This chiefly affects the limbs and is responsible for the loss of arm swinging when walking. In the face it appears as the classical mask with a fixed expression. The tongue, pharynx and vocal cords may be involved causing speech impairment. Rigidity of the respiratory muscles predisposes the patient to complications of bronchopneumonia.

Lack of initiation.

There may be *difficulty in passing water* or *urgency of micturition*.

Cases are selected for surgery, usually with an upper age limit of 65. A patient older than this is only considered if he is essentially unilaterally affected and has no physical or mental deterioration. The best results are obtained from the under-60 age-group with a slowly progressive form of the disease.

INVESTIGATIONS AND ASSESSMENTS

Plain X-ray films of the skull are taken. Electro-encephalography is performed.

The patient is assessed by the psychologist, the speech therapist, the occupational therapist and the physiotherapist.

Surgical treatment

Stereotaxic surgery is carried out under local anaesthetic in two stages, occasionally completed within the same day, but usually with a day of rest between.

The first stage consists of placing markers in the skull as a guide to the midsagittal plane of the brain.

The second stage consists of introducing Myodil (iophendylate injection) into the lateral and third ventricles to outline the anterior and posterior commissures. An electrode is passed through an occipital burr hole to the thalamus. Coagulation is carried out in the ventro-lateral nucleus of the thalamus to reduce tremor and in the globus pallidus to reduce rigidity (see Fig. 4/7, page 144).

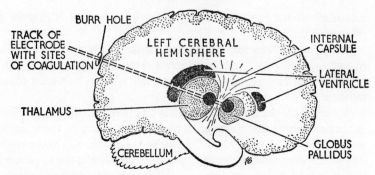

TRACK OF ELECTRODE WITH SITES OF COAGULATION

BURR HOLE

LEFT CEREBRAL HEMISPHERE

INTERNAL CAPSULE

LATERAL VENTRICLE

THALAMUS

GLOBUS PALLIDUS

CEREBELLUM

Fig. 4/7 Diagram showing position of burr hole in stereotaxic surgery for parkinsonism.

Stereotaxy is now being used mainly for the relief of tremor. Rigidity is being treated by the use of drugs, L-dopa being widely used.

Physiotherapy treatment

Breathing exercises must be practised hourly by the patient to reduce the risk of bronchopneumonia. Coughing may be difficult for the patient whose main symptom is rigidity.

The limbs freed from rigidity and tremor may require functional re-education. After loss of severe tremor the type of stabilizing exercises described for cerebellar ataxia (see page 140) help the patient to regain functional use of his limbs, particularly the upper limb. Full range joint mobility is rapidly regained when symptoms have been relieved.

The patient is allowed to sit up in bed the day after operation and to get up on the second postoperative day. Balance re-education is important for a patient with rigidity as the main symptom, and stabilization in sitting and standing is useful, the patient watching himself in a mirror. A patient with mainly tremor has little or no problem in regaining balance. Re-education of standing up and sitting down, walking, walking with arm swinging and turning round require patience and perseverance.

Standing up and sitting down, especially if a low chair is being used, is difficult for a parkinsonian patient. He must be taught to tuck his feet well underneath him, then use his hands on the edge of the chair to push his weight forward over his feet, then to straighten up. When sitting down he must be taught to feel for the chair and lower himself down gently.

Walking. To re-educate walking it must be impressed upon the patient to lift his feet and take a big step. Lifting the feet is over-emphasized at the outset, marking time on the spot prior to walking can be a useful preliminary followed by stepping over lines on the floor.

To re-educate arm-swinging while walking, poles are used, the patient holding one end of the pole in each hand, and the physiotherapist walking behind holding the other ends. Arm-swinging is done at first by the physiotherapist pushing the appropriate pole with the patient gradually taking over.

Turning. The great tendency is for the patient to jerk round suddenly when turning. He must be taught to do this slowly and lift his feet up. Re-education can begin with marking time on the spot, then turning round slowly still marking time.

Stairs. Apart from any difficulty with balance, the parkinsonian patient rarely has difficulty in going up or down stairs.

PROGRESSION OF TREATMENT

Progress can be made rapidly in the physiotherapy and occupational therapy departments once the patient is allowed up. About the third day he will be able to participate in some class work to music to assist re-education of balance and mobility. The class work can be increased on successive days to a full programme which includes exercises in sitting, standing and on the mat. Mat work to retrain rolling, sitting up, standing up to lying down and vice versa, and exercises on the mat to strengthen back extensor muscles are useful in that they help the patient regain his independence. He can then begin to move about in bed and get in and out of bed, activities which he will previously have found difficult.

EPILEPSY

Epilepsy can be described as a paroxysmal transitory disturbance of the functions of the brain which develops suddenly, ceases spontaneously, with a strong tendency to recurrence. Many varieties of epileptic attack exist, depending upon the site of origin, extent of spread and the nature of the disturbance of function.

Causes

Epilepsy may be caused by:
A local lesion in the brain, such as tumour or abscess, where epilepsy is the presenting feature;
Complication of a head injury due to a post-traumatic scar;
Hereditary predisposition; or
Unknown causes.

INVESTIGATIONS

Electro-encephalography. Recordings of the electrical activity of the brain can help to pinpoint the cause of epilepsy. If a focus can be determined, its nature can be investigated by other means.

Further appropriate measures will be selected according to the particular history of the patient.

Surgical treatment

Until recently surgery has only been indicated for certain selected cases and has been of value to a patient who has epilepsy as the presenting feature of a brain lesion, or a definite focus which gives rise to his epileptic attacks.

Surgical procedures vary with the type of lesion to be excised. Temporal lobe epilepsy may be treated by lobectomy. Increasingly stereotaxic procedures are being employed to treat certain forms of epilepsy, particularly a diffuse type which cannot be treated by drugs or cortical excision.

PHYSIOTHERAPY TREATMENT

A general programme of rehabilitation is carried out; defects are treated according to the symptoms.

INTRACTABLE PAIN

THALAMOTOMY

This procedure is briefly mentioned in the following chapter (p. 173) as it may follow various spinal procedures in an attempt to relieve pain.

Hypophysectomy

Certain types of cancer of the breast and prostate appear to be hormone dependent. A hormonal deprivation can produce some relief and lengthen survival. The pituitary gland produces hormones which influence other endocrine glands. An oophorectomy or adrenalectomy may be performed to assess whether the lesions are responsive to hormone control. If the patient has a dramatic relief of pain following one of these measures, hypophysectomy may then be indicated.

SURGICAL TREATMENT

There are several methods of either removing or destroying the pituitary gland. Removal can be done by a trans-oral, trans-nasal, or trans-sphenoidal approach. Destruction of the gland can be done by stereotaxic surgery.

Trans-frontal approach. This is performed under local anaesthetic through two burr holes situated near the mid-line at hair-line level.

Trans-ethmoidal approach. This requires a general anaesthetic. It is done through the inner angle of the eye bilaterally.

Trans-sphenoidal approach. This also requires a general anaesthetic. It is performed through the nose at the level of the inner angle of the eye bilaterally.

POSTOPERATIVE TREATMENT

Replacement drug therapy is given as required; some form of steroids are always necessary. Antibiotics are also given as meningitis is a possible complication. The patient is kept in isolation for the first few days until it has been established that no cerebrospinal fluid leak is apparent, another possible complication of this procedure. If no cerebrospinal fluid leak is present the patient is allowed to get up 24 hours after his operation.

PHYSIOTHERAPY TREATMENT

Breathing exercises begin immediately but the patient must be instructed not to blow his nose, and coughing must be achieved with the minimum strain, and only if secretions are present, due to the dangers of causing a cerebrospinal fluid leak.

Routine maintenance exercises, walking, etc. are allowed within the patient's tolerance, and bearing in mind the extent of the underlying lesion.

For Bibliography see end of Chapter 5.

CHAPTER 5

Surgery of the Spinal Cord

by M. C. BALFOUR, MCSP

ANATOMY AND PHYSIOLOGY

The spinal cord lies within the vertebral canal and extends from the foramen magnum to the lower border of the first lumbar vertebra. It is surrounded by meninges, as is the brain, and the cerebrospinal fluid circulates in the subarachnoid space between the pia mater and the arachnoid mater. This space descends as far as the second sacral vertebra. The blood supply is rich but complex and mainly derived from the posterior spinal arteries, the anterior spinal artery and segmental arteries which enter by the intervertebral foramina.

A pair of spinal nerves are given off at each segment of the cord, but due to the cord being shorter than the vertebral canal the segments do not tally with the numerically corresponding vertebrae. In the cervical region the segments lie one vertebra higher, while in the lumbar region the fifth lumbar nerve root is given off at the level of the twelfth thoracic vertebra. The mass of lumbar and sacral nerve roots given off at the lower end of the spinal cord is termed the cauda equina (see Fig. 5/1).

Each nerve root consists of an anterior motor root and a posterior sensory root, which pass separately through the dura mater, then unite. They then descend to the appropriate intervertebral foramen through which they issue. The course of these nerves is almost horizontal in the cervical region, but the lumbar nerves have a long vertical course before reaching their appropriate point of exit (see Fig. 5/1).

EFFECTS OF COMPRESSION ON THE SPINAL CORD

Any lesion in the region of the spinal cord which causes pressure affects the spinal cord and nerve roots in several ways:

148

Direct pressure interferes with conduction in the nerve roots and the spinal cord.

Pressure on the veins leads to oedema.

Pressure on the arteries leads to ischaemia.

Degeneration of nerve cells and fibres then takes place in the area.

The subarachnoid space becomes obstructed.

Compression of the cord can occur anywhere throughout its length and affects one or several segments. The pressure may affect both sides if the lesion is central, or one side more than the other if the lesion is lateral. Pressure on one side of the cord can gradually displace the cord and the nerve roots towards the opposite side of the vertebral canal, thus involving the healthy side. Motor and sensory symptoms can arise on both sides of the body if the lesion is central but can give a Brown-Séquard type of syndrome if the lesion is confined to one side of the cord.

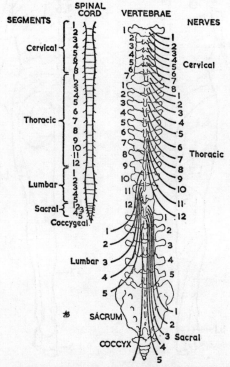

Fig. 5/1 Diagram showing spinal cord and spinal nerves.

BROWN-SEQUARD SYNDROME

On the side of the lesion the following occur:

There is loss of voluntary power due to the fact that the cerebrospinal tracts cross mainly in the medulla oblongata which lies well above the area of compression.

There is loss of muscle and joint sense, vibratory sense and tactile discrimination due to involvement of the posterior column.

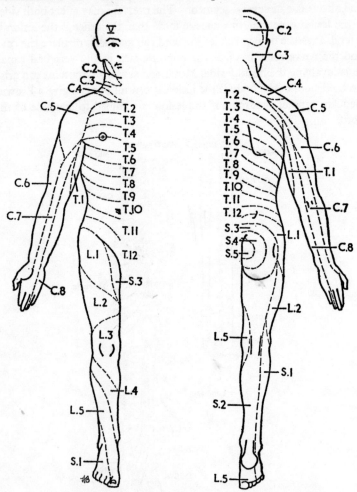

Fig. 5/2 Diagram showing the innervation of the skin.

Fibres of the lateral spinothalamic tract entering the cord just below
the level of the lesion are caught before they cross, causing a narrow
zone of pain and temperature loss immediately below the lesion.

On the opposite side of the lesion findings are as follows:

There is loss of pain and temperature sensations due to the destruction of the lateral spinothalamic tract, fibres of which enter the cord and
ascend for several segments, then cross. The upper level of the sensory
loss is therefore a few segments below the level of the lesion.

Fibres carrying light touch and tactile localization are partly crossed
and partly uncrossed, thus there is rarely loss of these sensibilities in a
unilateral lesion.

Pressure may be localized and affect only one nerve root, resulting in
pain, sensory loss and motor weakness in the distribution of this particular nerve root. In this area the sensory loss will be incomplete as
structures are rarely supplied by one nerve, but hyperaesthesia can be
present as an early feature.

Signs and symptoms arising from cord compression vary with the
degree of pressure, the exact position and extent of the lesion, and the
rate of progression.

Signs and symptoms of spinal cord compression

PAIN

This results from the irritant effect of the lesion on the nerve fibres. It
is usually the earliest symptom and has a segmental distribution (see
Fig. 5/2). It is a prominent feature in extramedullary lesions such as
neurinomas and extradural neoplasms and when nerve roots are involved
in cauda equina or disc lesions. Movements and increased intraspinal
pressure caused by coughing and sneezing will increase the pain. Tenderness on pressure may be present over the spinous processes supplied
by the nerves in the compressed area: this will be several vertebrae below the lesion. As pressure increases pain will decrease due to decreased
conductivity.

LOSS OF MOTOR POWER

This usually follows the sensory disturbance and takes the form of a
progressive weakness. The muscles affected are those supplied by the
segments of the cord which are being compressed and those supplied by
the segments below the lesion. If the lesion is unilateral the weakness

is present on the same side of the body; with a central lesion both sides are involved, but one side is usually more affected than the other.

MUSCLE TONE
At the level of the lesion tone will be diminished or lost, as this constitutes a lower motor neurone lesion. Below the level of the lesion there is an upper motor neurone lesion and tone will be increased as the pyramidal and extrapyramidal tracts are interrupted and the reflex arc is no longer inhibited by higher centres. In cauda equina lesions only a lower motor neurone lesion exists.

REFLEXES
As with muscle tone, reflexes are diminished at the level of the lesion and increased below the lesion.

SENSATION
This is diminished or lost below the lesion. Types of sensation involved will depend upon the site of the lesion as previously described. Involvement of the posterior column will affect kinaesthetic sensation, while the anterolateral column will affect pain and temperature. In cauda equina lesions sensory loss of all types is likely in the root distribution.

SPHINCTERS
These are not involved in the early stages but later precipitancy or difficulty with micturition develops and this may progress to retention of urine. Constipation is most usual with spinal neoplasms. Rectal incontinence rarely occurs.

AUTONOMIC DISTURBANCES
Sweating does not occur below the level of the lesion. Vasomotor disturbances occur, resulting in impaired circulation.

CEREBROSPINAL FLUID
If there is an obstruction of the subarachnoid space the chemical composition of this fluid changes. Its protein content is increased, which provides useful diagnostic information.

Mode of onset
The onset of symptoms is usually gradual when due to a spinal neoplasm, but rapid in malignant disease involving the vertebral column.

To clarify the effects of spinal cord compression at different levels the following signs and symptoms will be found:

COMPRESSION AT THE FIFTH CERVICAL SEGMENT
Muscle power and tone. Hypotonia and weakness will be present in the rhomboids, supra- and infraspinatus, deltoid, biceps, brachialis and brachioradialis. Spasticity and loss of voluntary power occurs in the other muscles of the upper limbs supplied by segments below the level of the lesion and in the trunk and legs.
Reflexes. The biceps and brachioradialis jerks will be diminished or lost; the triceps jerks and those of the lower extremities will be exaggerated. An extensor plantar response will be elicited on stimulation of the sole of the foot and clonus may be present at the ankle and knee. Superficial abdominal reflexes are absent.
Sensation. Loss occurs in the upper limbs apart from the lateral aspect, and over the trunk and lower limbs.
Sphincters. The bladder and bowel functions are disturbed.

COMPRESSION OF THE CAUDA EQUINA
Muscle power and tone. A flaccid paralysis occurs in muscles supplied by the compressed nerve roots. The muscles of the leg and foot are likely to be more involved than those of the hip and knee, due to the longer course within the vertebral canal of the nerves supplying them.
Reflexes. These are diminished according to the nerve roots involved. Compression of the fourth lumbar nerve root will cause loss of the knee jerk, and compression of the first sacral nerve root will cause loss of the ankle jerk.
Sensation. Some scattered loss occurs but it is not likely to be complete.
Sphincters. The bladder and bowel function will be disturbed.

Special investigations

After careful clinical examination special investigations are carried out to establish the exact site, extent and nature of the lesion.
X-rays. Plain films are usually necessary.
Lumbar puncture is carried out to obtain specimens of cerebrospinal fluid for diagnostic purposes and to establish if there is a block of the subarachnoid space.

Myelography. Myodil or air, usually the former, is introduced via a lumbar puncture needle and guided to the appropriate region. Where a complete spinal block is present, Myodil (iophendylate) may be introduced via a cisternal puncture into the cisterna magna and allowed to flow down to outline the upper level of the lesion. The Myodil is removed at the end of the examination as it tends to act as an irritant.

Lumbar radiculography. A water-soluble contrast medium such as Conray 280 or Dimer X is now being used to investigate lumbar nerve roots. Following this examination the patient has to remain erect (seated or propped up in bed) for six hours in order to prevent the contrast medium reaching the spinal cord, to which it is very irritating.

CONDITIONS SUITABLE FOR SURGERY

Neoplasms. Primary neoplasms arise from the cord, the meninges or the sheaths of the spinal nerves.

Secondary neoplasms usually involve the vertebral bodies and may cause compression of the neural elements, that is the spinal cord and nerve roots.

Infections such as an epidural abscess can only be dealt with by surgical intervention.

Protruded intervertebral discs.

Degenerative lesions such as cervical spondylosis require surgery to relieve existing symptoms and prevent further deterioration.

Intractable pain may be caused by lesions which may be outside the central nervous system.

Congenital deformities, e.g. spina bifida (see *Neurology for Physiotherapists,* Chapter XI).

Spinal neoplasms

NEOPLASMS OF THE SPINAL CORD

Spinal neoplasms occur in any age-group, but are rather more common between the ages of 20 and 60. The sexes are affected equally.

They are classified as extradural (those which lie outside the membranes surrounding the cord), and intradural (those which lie inside the membranes). The intradural type is further classified into extramedullary, which do not enter the spinal cord (such as the meningiomas and neurinomas), and intramedullary, which arise in the substance of the cord (such as the ependymomas).

The onset of symptoms with these neoplasms is usually very slow and may extend over a period of years.

NEOPLASMS OF THE VERTEBRAL COLUMN

The commonest type of neoplasm is a secondary carcinoma which usually attacks the vertebral body. The primary lesion is often in the breast in women and the prostate gland and the lung in men. Sarcomas are examples of primary neoplasms. The secondary carcinomas grow very rapidly, giving rise to acute spinal cord compression, and require emergency treatment.

Infections of the spine

These include epidural abscesses and tuberculosis (Pott's paraplegia).

EPIDURAL ABSCESS

This can be caused by osteomyelitis of the vertebral column, infections in the body such as the lungs and peritoneal cavity, skin infections of the back and lumbar puncture. Tuberculosis of the spine may also produce a 'cold' abscess.

The size of the lesion can vary from a very small localized area to one involving the entire length of the cord. The onset of symptoms may be acute, sub-acute or chronic. If acute, emergency surgery will be required. Once pressure on the spinal cord has been relieved, antibiotics are introduced by means of a drain to control the infection.

TUBERCULOSIS (Pott's paraplegia)

This usually occurs in children and young adults, but no age-group is exempt. The infective process usually begins in the body of a vertebra and spreads to adjacent vertebral bodies which leads to their collapse. An angular deformity of the spine is thus produced. This deformity, an associated tuberculous abscess or interference with the vascular supply of sub-adjacent segments, can disturb spinal cord function and a paraplegia may develop.

SURGICAL TREATMENT

To relieve compression of the spinal cord caused by neoplasms and abscesses, a laminectomy is usually carried out at the appropriate levels. This decompresses the spinal cord without disturbing the stability of the vertebral column.

Laminectomy

A fairly long mid-line incision is made and the back muscles stripped from the spinous processes and the laminae, which are then removed, the number removed depending on the extent of the lesion. Neoplasms of the extramedullary type are removed entirely or as far as possible. The intramedullary type which invade the cord substance may not be removed entirely. The cord will be incised and as much material as possible removed, the dura being left open to effect a further decompression.

POSTOPERATIVE TREATMENT

On return from theatre the patient is nursed in side lying with a pillow supporting his back, his underneath leg straight and the top leg flexed at hip and knee and supported by two pillows, one under the thigh and one under the leg. To prevent pressure sores two-hourly turns are essential, the patient going from side to front, from front to his other side. If there are signs of bladder involvement prior to operation, a catheter will be draining the bladder, which is maintained until bladder function returns or an automatic bladder trained.

If there is loss of sensation the patient will be nursed on pillow packs to prevent the development of pressure sores. Great care must be taken to ensure that the coverings on the packs are kept unwrinkled. Positioning and turning procedures are as previously described. A bedcage is used to keep the weight of the bedclothes off the feet and a firm support placed at the bottom of the bed to maintain the feet at right angles, thus preventing a foot drop.

For a lesion of the cervical spine, with loss of power and sensation in the upper limbs, careful positioning of the arms is necessary to ensure that the elbows do not develop flexion contractures. A roll of Sorbo rubber in the hand keeps the fingers in a functional position and the wrist is in slight extension. If necessary a pillow can be used to keep the upper arm away from the chest wall.

With an extensive laminectomy the patient may find lying on the back uncomfortable until the tenth day, when sutures will be removed, or partly so, and the wound feels less tender.

GENERAL PHYSIOTHERAPY PRINCIPLES

Bearing in mind the principles outlined in the previous chapter, only specific points of postoperative physiotherapy treatment will follow each condition.

Physiotherapy treatment

BREATHING EXERCISES AND COUGHING

When a lesion involves the intercostal and abdominal muscles, the diaphragm is the only remaining muscle of respiration. The patient must be encouraged to practise breathing exercises regularly to reduce the danger of bronchopneumonia. Coughing will be reduced in force and can be assisted by pushing up under the diaphragm with the hand. Where voluntary power allows, the patient is taught to do this for himself, and if he is unable to do so the nurses are taught how to assist him.

MAINTENANCE EXERCISES

These are carried out where possible to maintain circulation. If no voluntary power is present, passive movements are carried out twice daily.

CAREFUL POSITIONING AND PASSIVE MOVEMENTS

These are necessary to prevent contractures. When the arms are involved it is important to retain full range shoulder movements, full extension of the elbow and prevent tightening of the wrist and finger flexors. Flexion and extension of the metacarpophalangeal joints and a full stretch on the web of the thumb are important. In the lower limb it is important to retain full extension of the hip and knee and the ability to get the feet to a right angle. Hamstring muscles should not be allowed to become tight. During the first few postoperative days no hamstring stretching should be given as it might produce pain due to stretching of the nerve roots and a pull on the meninges. After approximately one week gentle hamstring stretching can be commenced in a small range, gradually increasing until the leg, with the foot at 90° to the leg, can be raised to a right angle to the body.

RETURN OF FUNCTION

This is encouraged by means of facilitation techniques.

STATIC CONTRACTIONS

Static abdominal and back muscle contractions can begin on the first day. Active abdominal work can begin when the sutures are removed and active back extension is begun gently approximately on the third day.

SHOULDER GIRDLE STRENGTHENING

This may be started immediately with arm exercises. If the incision is a high one care must be taken that there is no pull on the wound. Spring resistance can be given if there is no danger of pulling on the wound, and can be commenced when the patient's back is comfortable. When there is gross loss of voluntary power in the lower limbs it is most important to develop the muscles of the shoulder girdle and latissimus dorsi as they will be required for lifting and when walking with crutches.

BALANCE RE-EDUCATION

This begins when the patient is allowed to get up approximately after the fourth day. It is advisable to get him to tolerate an upright position in bed before he gets up. Balance re-education can begin by sitting the patient over the edge of the bed with the feet supported on the floor or on a stool, then in a wheelchair. In the early stages a mirror is useful to help the patient regain his balance, especially if he has sensory loss. When he has gained balance in a wheelchair and on the edge of the bed, mat work can be started and balance in long sitting.

Mat work. The patient must practise sitting up, rolling from side to side and rolling on to his front, getting into a kneeling position and balancing in this position. He must practise moving across and up and down the mat using his arms to lift his buttocks. Hip raising and balancing in this position helps to regain stability. Back extension, hip extension and hamstring exercises can be given in prone lying. Crawling in all directions, free and against resistance, helps to strengthen hip muscles. Further balance re-education is done in kneeling and half-kneeling and practice in getting from this position on and off a chair or stool is the next progression.

Wheelchair. If the patient has a gross or permanent disability a wheelchair will be necessary to enable him to become independent. Each patient is measured and a chair and Sorbo cushion is ordered to his specific requirements. The patient must be taught to control and manoeuvre his chair. When his balance and arm power are adequate the patient is taught to transfer himself from bed to wheelchair and from wheelchair to bed. Later he is taught to get from his chair to the mat and *vice versa*.

RE-EDUCATION OF WALKING

Re-education of walking commences with balance in standing. This usually begins with the patient between parallel bars with a mirror in front of him. When the patient can balance satisfactorily, walking re-education is commenced. The ability to progress along these lines depends on the degree of voluntary power loss. When the patient is ready to stand, various aids may be necessary. As a temporary measure plaster back slabs to keep the knees straight may be used. If gross muscle weakness persists calipers will be needed. The calipers are made to measure with a corset top, jointed at the knee, and a toe-raising device if necessary. If weakness is only in the anterior tibial muscles below-knee calipers may be needed.

The type of gait taught depends upon the level of the lesion. This may be four-point if the lesion is at or below the tenth thoracic segment, or swing-to, for lesions above this level. Once walking has become controlled in the parallel bars the patient can progress to using elbow crutches, beginning with one bar and one crutch, then balancing on both crutches, then to walking. A mirror can be used at the beginning of each progression until the patient gains the correct idea of balance and gait. If the patient uses a wheelchair he must be taught how to stand up and sit down using his crutches.

Stairs. The patient can be re-educated to use the stairs by using a banister rail and one elbow crutch. Going up the stairs the patient puts his crutch up on the step first then jumps his feet up. Coming down he swings his legs down one step then brings his crutch down.

When a patient has voluntary control of his hips and knees, elbow crutches are not necessary. He can walk with the aid of quadruped or tripod sticks in initial stages, and may be progressed to walking sticks when his balance and confidence improve. When going upstairs he uses the banister rail and one stick. He puts his stick up first, then his right foot, the stick goes up to the next step, followed by his left foot. Coming down he puts his stick down first, then his right foot to the same step, his stick down to the next step followed by his left foot.

A patient with sensory loss. Measures taken to prevent pressure sores developing in the early stages of postoperative care have already been pointed out (p. 156) and nursing care has been directed to this end. If beds become wet they are immediately changed and the patient sponged and dried. Time must be taken to explain to the patient what this sensory loss means to him and he must be taught to look after his skin to prevent any sores developing. He should be instructed in the following points:

He must examine his skin carefully each day, using a mirror where necessary.

A hot-water bottle must never be used.

Special care must be taken when cutting toe- and fingernails. If there is a tendency to ingrowing toenails the skin should be massaged away from the nail. If the nail does grow into the skin, suppuration may occur and the nail may need to be removed.

If thick hard skin develops on hands and feet it should be softened with cream or olive oil and removed.

Bath water must be checked for temperature before the patient gets into the bath. A piece of sponge rubber in the bottom of the bath prevents the patient getting bruised. Cold water should be run into the bath first in case the heat of the bath itself causes a burn.

Warning should be given with regard to sitting near fires and radiators and in direct sunlight.

In cold weather the feet must be kept warm to prevent chilblains developing.

For patients with loss of sensation in the hands, cups should have a protective covering or holder and a cigarette holder must be used if the patient smokes.

When sitting in a chair he must frequently lift his buttocks off the cushion to relieve pressure. This is taught immediately he starts using his wheelchair. If arm power is inadequate a physiotherapist, or nurse, must lift the patient regularly until his balance will allow him to move sufficiently from hip to hip to relieve pressure.

If the patient wishes to sit in an ordinary armchair he must make sure it has a soft seat.

Shoes must be chosen carefully to ensure they do not produce sores; soft leather with no toecaps are advisable, and a half-size larger and wider fitting than previously worn.

If a pressure sore develops the quickest way to heal this is to keep the patient in bed and nurse him in a position which will keep all

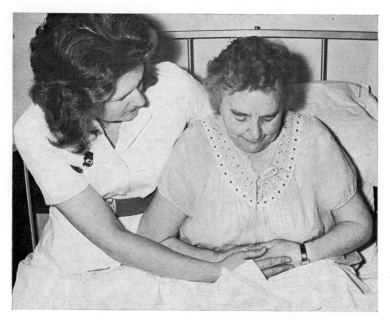

3/1 A patient being assisted to cough, while in bed (*see p.* 86)

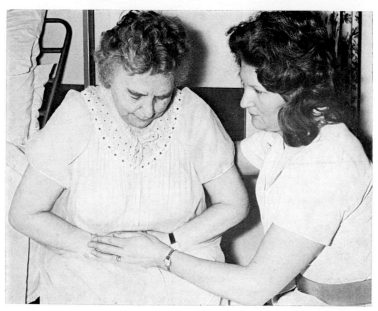

3/2 A patient being assisted to cough, while sitting in a chair
(*see p.* 86)

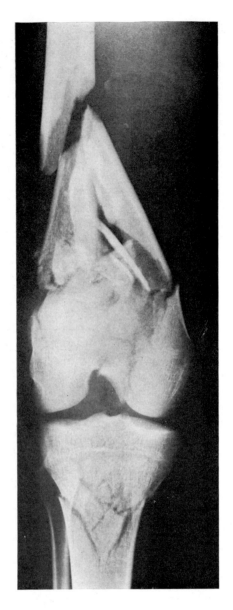

10/1 Comminuted fractures of upper
tibia and lower femur

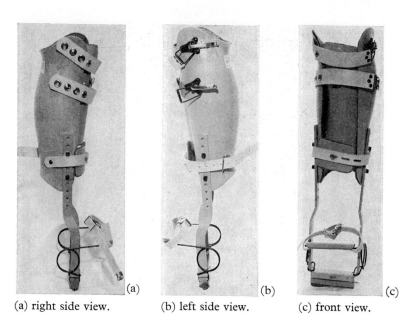

(a) right side view.   (b) left side view.   (c) front view.

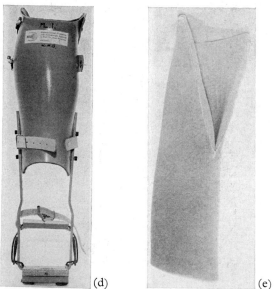

(d) back view. (e) protective sock worn inside the caliper (*see p.* 269)

10/2 Special caliper used with the A.O. method of treating fractures of the tibia.

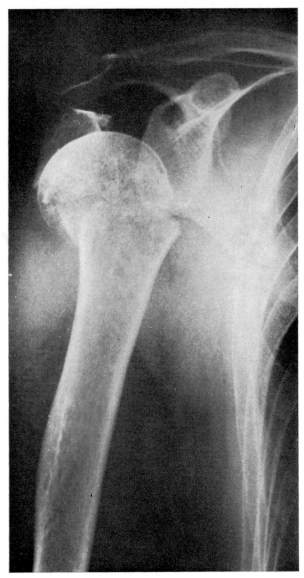

11/1 Impacted fracture of neck of humerus (*see* p. 274)

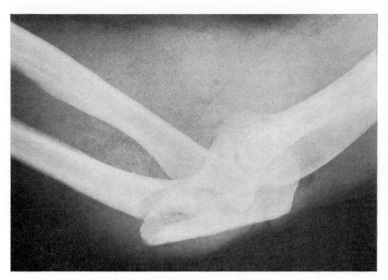

11/2 (a) Monteggia's fracture of radius and ulna.

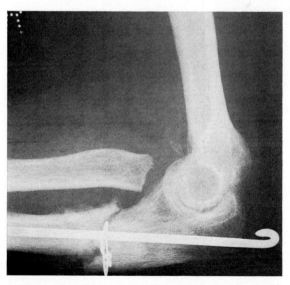

11/2 (b) After head of radius removed, ulna fixed with a Rush nail (*see p. 264*)

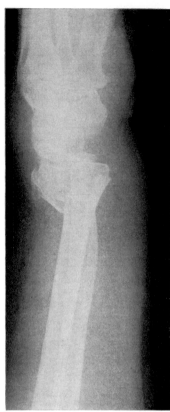

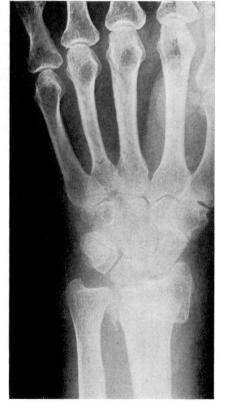

11/3 Colles' fracture of the
wrist (*see p.* 280) above and right

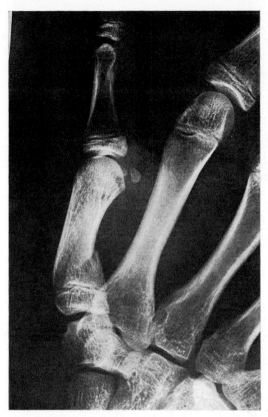

11/4 Bennett's fracture of the first metacarpal
(*see p.* 280)

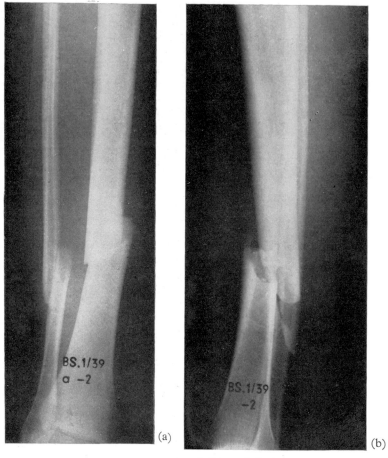

(a)

(b)

11/5 (a) and (b) Fractures of shafts of tibia and fibula.

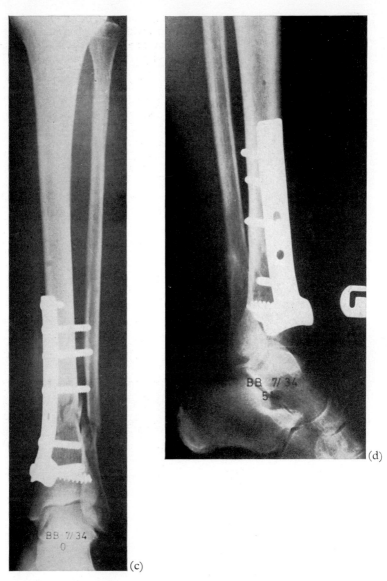

(c)

(d)

11/5 (c) and (d) Fractures treated by compression plating (*see p.* 286)

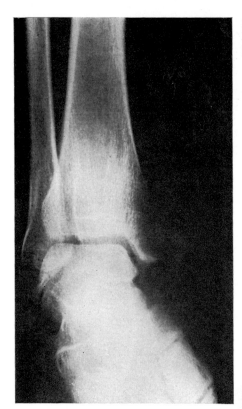

11/6 Fracture of lateral malleo-
lus, with no displacement of
joint mortice (*see p.* 286)

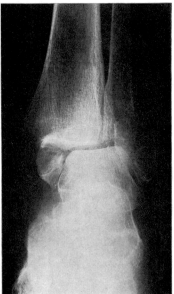

11/7 Pott's fracture of both malleoli, with
disruption of joint mortice (*see p.* 286)

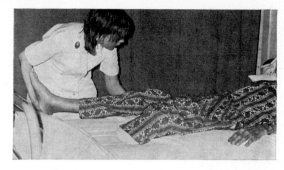

12/1 Extensor work for unaffected leg, showing strong isometric work to emphasize supportive function (*see p.* 301)

12/2 'Bridging', extension at pelvis (*see p.* 301)

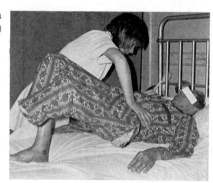

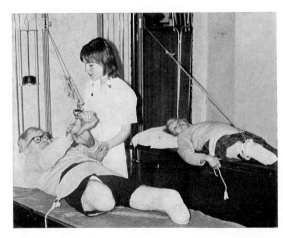

12/3 Weight and pulley work. Left: bilateral upper limb extension for trunk.
Right: extension, abduction, medial rotation pattern of right leg (*see p.* 301)

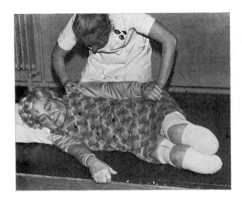

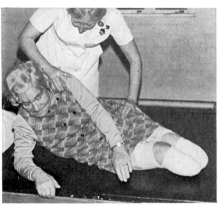

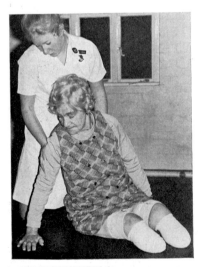

12/4–6 Rolling to sitting sequence
with guided resistance (*see p.* 301)

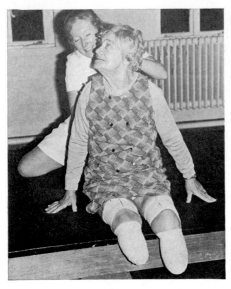

12/7 Resisted sitting
balance (*see p.* 301)

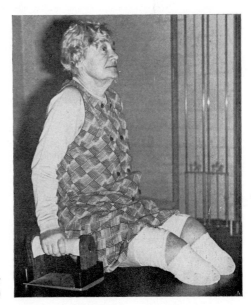

12/8 Extensor 'push-ups' for
upper limbs (*see p.* 301)

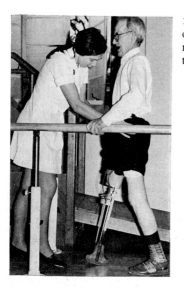

12/9 Right above-knee amputee on pylon, physiotherapist giving resistance at pelvis for weight transference (*see p.* 305)

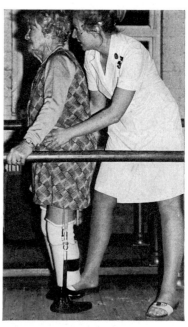

12/11 Resistance at pelvis to emphasize hip extension. Note rocker bases extend posteriorly to prevent patient losing balance backwards, particularly important if there is any hip flexion contracture (*see p.* 307)

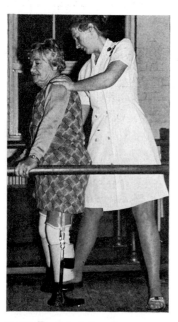

12/10 Double below-knee amputee on pylons, resisted standing balance in parallel bars (*see p.* 307)

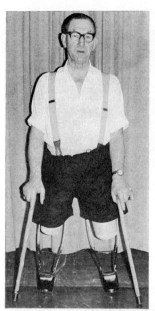

12/12 Double above-knee amputee on short rocker pylons. Note necessity of wide base (*see p.* 307)

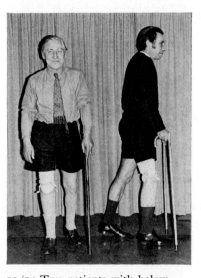

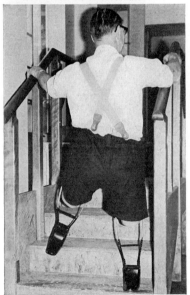

12/13 Climbing stairs, rocker is placed on edge of step and patient extends the hip on that side as he pulls with his hands on the rails (*see p.* 307)

12/14 Two patients with below-knee amputations wearing patellar tendon bearing prostheses. Note that control of the prosthesis depends entirely upon the hip and knee joints and muscles, particularly the quadriceps and hamstrings

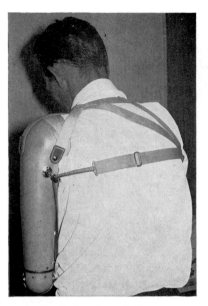

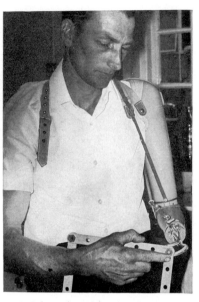

12/15 Posterior view of above-elbow prosthesis showing leather operating cord (inferior) attached to appendages. Protraction of scapulae to operate terminal device (*see p.* 310)

12/16 Anterior view showing strap to operate elbow lock

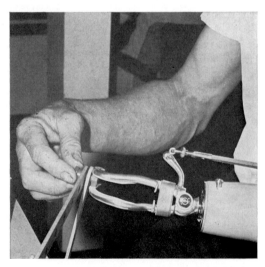

12/17 Close-up of split hook (*see p.* 310)

pressure from the area. He should not be allowed to get up again until the sore is adequately healed.

INTERVERTEBRAL DISCS

Intervertebral discs are found between the bodies of the movable vertebrae and extend from the second cervical vertebra to the lumbo-sacral junction. In the lumbar region they are much thicker and shaped to the lumbar curve. Each vertebral body is covered with hyaline cartilage and the disc, consisting of an outer fibrocartilaginous annulus fibrosus and an inner gelatinous nucleus pulposus, is sandwiched between. The annulus fibrosus is weakest posterolaterally where it is inadequately supported by the spinous ligaments. This is where it becomes thinned as a result of trauma and may rupture completely if the initial trauma is sufficiently severe.

When the annulus fibrosus becomes thinned the results are as follows:

The nucleus pulposus bulges at the weakened point. The nerve root passing down the vertebral canal to emerge through the appropriate

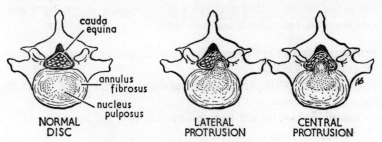

Fig. 5/3 Lumbar disc herniations.

intervertebral foramen becomes stretched over this bulge. This causes pain due to irritation with subsequent compression, causing loss of sensation and motor power.

The annulus fibrosus may rupture and allow the nucleus to pass through the opening in the spinous ligaments to lie in the vertebral canal.

Occasionally the nucleus pulposus may herniate in the mid-line giving rise to symptoms similar to a spinal cord neoplasm in the cervical region and a cauda equina lesion in the lumbar region (see Fig. 5/3).

LUMBAR DISC HERNIATIONS

The lumbar region is the commonest site of a disc herniation. The highest incidence is between the fourth and fifth lumbar vertebrae and the fifth lumbar and the first sacral vertebrae.

General signs and symptoms of a lumbar disc herniation

Pain. Backache may be the presenting feature, but the patient usually complains of pain in the distribution of the sciatic nerve. Bending and straining will increase the pain.

The lumbar curve is obliterated and the paravertebral muscles are in spasm.

Scoliosis. Some degree of scoliosis may occur, usually away from the side of the lesion, which relieves pressure on the nerve root.

Straight leg-raising is decreased.

Sensory changes. These are usually found over the lateral aspect of the calf and heel.

Depressed tendon reflexes. The ankle jerk is diminished or lost if the first sacral nerve root is compressed. The knee jerk is diminished or lost if the fourth lumbar nerve root is compressed. These signs and symptoms are intermittent and will recur with any fresh trauma.

SYNDROME OF A DISC PROTRUSION BETWEEN THE FOURTH AND FIFTH LUMBAR VERTEBRAE

Pain, down the posterolateral aspect of the thigh and lateral aspect of the leg, to the ankle.

Sensory changes, usually pins and needles, over the lateral aspect of the leg.

Motor weakness, involving extensor hallucis longus first, but may eventually involve all the other dorsiflexors.

SYNDROME OF A DISC PROTRUSION BETWEEN THE FIFTH LUMBAR AND FIRST SACRAL VERTEBRAE

Pain, down the posterolateral aspect of the thigh and lateral aspect of the leg extending to the outer border of the foot.

Sensory changes, usually over the outer border of the foot and little toe, which may extend over the foot and involve the other toes.

The ankle jerk is depressed.

Motor weakness, involving the plantarflexors.

Conservative treatment

The patient should rest in bed until the symptoms abate. He must lie on a firm mattress or have fracture boards under the mattress to ensure that his spine is adequately supported.

Continuous lumbar traction can be used to separate the vertebral bodies in the hope that the nucleus pulposus will return to its normal position.

A plaster jacket may be used.

Physiotherapy may be given.

Indications for surgical treatment

The relief of symptoms by surgical means becomes necessary when conservative treatment no longer affords relief, when progressive nerve root involvement appears, namely weakness and sensory loss, and/or when there are signs of cauda equina compression and bladder involvement. Emergency surgery is required in this instance to prevent irreparable damage to the spinal cord.

SPECIAL INVESTIGATIONS

Lumbar radiculography. This is now being used as a routine measure.

Surgical treatment

This treatment is aimed at the removal of the nucleus pulposus, or the ruptured part of the annulus fibrosus. The method of approach depends on the site and size of the protrusion.

Several operative techniques can be used to remove a lumbar disc herniation, all requiring a fairly long mid-line incision, to expose the spinous processes and laminae. The following procedures can then be carried out:

Fenestration. At the site of the disc protrusion the ligament is removed between the laminae, then a small portion of the lamina of the vertebrae above and below the protrusion is removed and the nerve root retracted. The exposed protrusion is then incised and as much as possible of the nucleus pulposus gouged out.

Laminectomy. This procedure is used when both sides of the disc space require exploration, usually in the case of a centrally protruded disc. The spinous process and both laminae are removed at the appropriate level and the disc protrusion dealt with as before.

POSTOPERATIVE TREATMENT

Nursing care is of paramount importance during the first few postoperative days. The patient is nursed in the side-lying position previously described and turned two-hourly, going from side to front to his other side, all pillows being removed to facilitate turning. In the early postoperative period the patient uses a bedpan in prone lying to avoid flexion of the spine.

Physiotherapy treatment

A wide variety of postoperative routines exists, each surgeon having his own ideas as to how the patient should be progressed. Each patient presents an individual problem and any routine must be adjusted to suit his capabilities. The general principles which apply to all routines are firstly to limit all exercises to the pain-free range of movement of the patient, and secondly, when giving mobilizing exercises, never force a particular movement.

METHODS

Breathing exercises and coughing. The patient may require encouragement if his wound is painful. Firm pressure over the wound from the physiotherapist's hand and instructions to tighten his abdominal muscles as he coughs are helpful measures. Breathing exercises should be practised hourly.

Maintenance exercises confined to foot and knee movements are practised hourly by the patient. Hip movements in a small range of flexion and extension to mid-line can begin on the first day, together with static abdominal work. Abduction of the hip and increased range of flexion with extension beyond the mid-line and straight leg raising follow as progressions of hip movement.

Static contractions of back extensor muscles are usually commenced on the *third* day. At this stage the patient can begin lying on his back for short periods. Care must be taken with his posture so he is taught to appreciate when he is lying in a straight line. Active extension usually follows on the fourth day, the number of times the exercises are repeated and the strength of the exercises are gradually increased.

Any specific muscle weakness is re-educated by means of facilitation techniques.

The re-education of posture in lying is progressed to re-education of posture in standing. The surgeon decides when the patient should be allowed to get up, which will be between the first and fifth day. Before the patient gets up it is advisable to elevate the bed to allow him to adjust to a more upright position. It must be noted that the entire bed is elevated: the patient is not placed in a sitting position. The patient is taught to lie on his side at the edge of the bed, put his feet over the edge and sit up keeping his back straight. His posture is corrected as soon as he stands up and he is re-educated in walking when necessary. On returning to bed he sits on the edge of the bed and with his back straight lies down on his side, bringing his legs into bed as he does so. Some patients may find it easier to get out of bed from a prone lying position. To do this he moves himself into a diagonal position across the bed, when his feet touch the floor he then pushes himself into an upright position keeping his back straight. Getting into bed, he keeps his back straight and lowers the top of his body by bending from the hips, then lifts his legs into bed. The patient is encouraged to get up for short periods and walk about.

The following instructions should be given:

A hard upright chair must be used and he must keep his back straight when sitting down and standing up. The sitting position should only be used at mealtimes and for short periods as it is usually an uncomfortable one.

When picking objects up from the floor he should be taught to go down on one knee keeping his back straight.

No lifting should be attempted.

If his back becomes uncomfortable he should lie down and rest.

Mobilization of the spine begins after the sutures are removed, usually the tenth day. Side flexion, rotation and forward flexion are all encouraged. Hydrotherapy is a useful means by which mobility can be encouraged.

When the patient is ready for discharge home he should be given a scheme of exercises to practise daily and instructed to continue these exercises for an indefinite period. The surgeon will decide when the patient is able to assume his normal activities and if any change of employment is necessary.

CERVICAL DISC HERNIATIONS

Herniation of the nucleus pulposus in the cervical region is less common than in the lumbar region. The usual sites of herniation are between the fifth and sixth, and sixth and seventh cervical vertebrae. This is probably due to the greater stress at these levels, as they lie at the point where the free mobility of the cervical spine is changing to the relative immobility of the thoracic spine. Herniation can occur spontaneously or as a result of trauma. The protrusion is usually in a posterolateral direction, but a central herniation can occur giving symptoms of spinal cord compression.

Signs and symptoms

Pain occurs in the neck on movement and may be severe. Referred pain in the distribution of the compressed nerve root is also present.

There is rigidity of the neck muscles.

The head may be slightly flexed to the side of the lesion.

Muscle wasting occurs in the motor distribution of the compressed nerve root, but severe loss of muscle power is not usual.

Sensory changes may occur over the appropriate dermatome.

Tendon reflexes innervated by the compressed nerve are diminished or lost.

Conservative treatment

Neck traction may be given to relieve pressure on the nerve root, and the neck immobilized by use of a collar.

Surgical treatment

When conservative measures fail to relieve the symptoms, surgical intervention is indicated. This will be described at the end of this section, p. 169.

CERVICAL SPONDYLOSIS

Degeneration of the intervertebral discs with the formation of osteophytes, especially at the intervertebral joints, are the pathological changes giving rise to cervical spondylosis. These intervertebral joints are the articulations between the bodies of the cervical vertebrae, they lie at the lateral margins of the intervertebral discs and are sometimes known as the joints of Lushka.

Individuals most affected are those in the middle and older age-groups. The most common site of the lesion is between the fifth and sixth and sixth and seventh vertebrae. Compression of the nerve roots can occur on one or both sides, at one or several levels.

The disease presents in two main patterns: cervical spondylosis with brachialgia, when the nerve roots are involved, and cervical myelopathy when there is spinal cord involvement.

Cervical spondylosis with brachialgia

The history of symptoms is very variable and onset of radicular symptoms may be acute, sub-acute or insidious. An acute onset of symptoms which involves one nerve root closely resembles an acute cervical disc herniation. An insidious onset is characterized by burning and tingling sensations down the arm.

SIGNS AND SYMPTOMS

A general picture of the signs and symptoms is as follows:

Burning and tingling sensations are often accompanied by pain radiating down the arm and into the fingers, the little and ring finger usually being involved. These symptoms tend to be worse at night.

The ability to appreciate light touch and pinprick is diminished in the dermatomes supplied by the compressed nerve roots.

There is localized tenderness of muscles supplied by the affected nerves.

Kinaesthetic sensation is impaired.

Slight muscle wasting and hypotonia are present in the muscles supplied by the compressed nerve roots.

Tendon reflexes are diminished or lost.

Neck movements are limited but relatively pain-free.

Local tenderness in the neck is elicited on pressure.

CONSERVATIVE TREATMENT

This is by immobilization by use of a collar, and physiotherapy including traction, heat, massage and exercises.

Cervical myelopathy

SIGNS AND SYMPTOMS

The patient presents with a progressive, spastic paraparesis with variable sensory loss, which cannot be differentiated from the signs and symptoms of a spinal cord neoplasm. Findings therefore are as for cervical cord compression (p. 148).

SURGICAL MANAGEMENT

This is designed to relieve nerve roots and spinal cord compression by the degenerated disc and osteophyte formation. The anterior approach is superseding the posterior approach but both will be mentioned.

If the lesion is lateral and the nerve root only is involved, a posterior approach with a hemilaminectomy is usually undertaken.

If myelopathy is present two alternative approaches are possible: a wide decompression of the spinal cord by means of a laminectomy, or an anterior cervical decompression and fusion.

POSTOPERATIVE TREATMENT FOLLOWING HEMILAMINECTOMY OR LAMINECTOMY

The patient is nursed in side lying, until his neck wound becomes less tender and he can tolerate back lying.

PHYSIOTHERAPY TREATMENT

Following hemilaminectomy

If this involves one level only, the patient will be allowed to get up between the fifth and seventh days. Static neck exercises, particularly for the neck extensor muscles, may begin about the same time. Active neck and shoulder exercises follow when sutures are removed, approximately on the tenth day. Any muscle weakness is re-educated by facilitation techniques.

Following laminectomy

If several laminae have been removed the patient will remain in bed until the tenth day. Static neck exercises begin on the seventh day. Some surgeons prefer a cervical collar to be fitted before the patient is allowed to get up, and he continues to wear it for a variable period of time. Once sutures have been removed gentle neck and shoulder exercises may be done without the collar, and particular attention must be paid to the patient's head and shoulder posture.

ANTERIOR CERVICAL DECOMPRESSION AND FUSION

This operation has been found to be more effective than a laminectomy.

The anatomy of the cervical region is such that a posterior approach by means of a laminectomy requires retraction of the spinal cord in order to reach the disc protrusion and the osteophytes. Manipulation of the spinal cord may upset its blood supply with disastrous results. The posterior approach can also weaken the neck muscles and subluxation may occur as a postoperative complication.

The anterior approach is a much safer procedure. Discs and osteophytes can be completely excised and the spine fused to prevent further osteophyte formation. Indications for operation are:

disease of the cervical discs when conservative measures have failed to relieve the symptoms;

certain types of injury to the cervical spine due to hyperextension and hyperflexion of the neck; and

certain neoplasms and infective processes such as tuberculosis of the cervical spine.

Surgical procedure

The patient lies supine with 25 pounds (11·3 kg) head traction. An incision is made in a skin crease in the right carotid triangle, exposing the anterior aspect of the spinal column from the second cervical to the first thoracic vertebral body. At the appropriate level a hole, half an inch (13 mm) in diameter is drilled through the disc and adjacent vertebral bodies until the posterior longitudinal ligament is reached. The debris of disc material and osteophytes is removed and a plug of bone, usually from the left iliac crest, inserted in the hole.

POSTOPERATIVE TREATMENT

The patient returns from theatre in a supine position with a Sorbo wing collar, which maintains the head in a mid-line position, allowing no lateral movement or rotation. A check X-ray is done early on the first day and if this is satisfactory the patient is then allowed to get up wearing a cervical collar. The collar is worn for three or four weeks if only one or two disc spaces have been fused, and for six weeks if three discs have been treated. A further X-ray however is done before the decision is made to discard the collar.

Postoperative physiotherapy

Breathing exercises and coughing. The patient practises his breathing exercises hourly.

Maintenance exercises. Particular attention is given to the left lower limb, especially hip movements. The patient needs encouragement to begin hip movements and quadriceps contractions, as the hip area is stiff and painful following the removal of bone from the ilium. Gentle full-range movements of the shoulder joints must be encouraged. Maintenance exercises must be practised hourly.

Re-education of any muscle weakness is carried out by means of facilitation techniques.

Walking re-education is often necessary, especially if the lower limbs were spastic due to spinal cord compression. Walking between parallel bars with the aid of a mirror helps the patient to appreciate where to place his feet. Later some type of walking aid may be necessary to make him independent.

CARE OF THE PATIENT'S NECK

The aims are to strengthen neck and shoulder muscles, and to regain mobility.

Methods. Static contractions of the neck and shoulder muscles are begun approximately on the third day with the patient in a supine position. When he is out of bed wearing a collar he is encouraged to practise these static contractions at regular intervals.

When the collar is removed between three to six weeks from the date of operation, active neck and shoulder exercises are given.

INTRACTABLE PAIN

Intractable pain describes a chronic severe pain which persists after the primary lesion has been treated. This type of pain serves no useful purpose and the patient's suffering can be relieved only by constant narcotic therapy. This becomes progressively less effective and there is constant danger of addiction to the drugs used.

Pain cannot be measured and has different characteristics depending on its origin. Innumerable factors can influence it, among the most important are the patient's personality, intelligence and emotional maturity. A careful assessment is thus essential before surgical measures are undertaken to relieve pain. When surgery is used for this purpose it is an indication that no further treatment is possible for the original disease.

Lesions giving rise to intractable pain are largely carcinomas outside the central nervous system. Herpes zoster, operational scars, amputation stump neuromas, phantom limb pain, and some cord lesions are non-malignant causes.

Surgical treatment

POSTERIOR RHIZOTOMY

The appropriate posterior spinal nerve roots are sectioned between the spinal cord and the posterior spinal ganglion, on the same side of the body as the intractable pain is appreciated. Due to the overlap of the sensory supply from one dermatome to another, it is necessary to section at least two sensory roots above and below the area in which pain is localized by the patient. This operation is carried out for post-herpetic pain and painful scars, but after a period of time the intractable pain tends to recur. It is of no use for limb pain, as it destroys muscle and joint sensation, which would give rise to a severe disability.

SPINOTHALAMIC CORDOTOMY

Fibres of the lateral spinothalamic tract are divided on the opposite side of the body to that on which the pain is appreciated. To achieve a permanent result this procedure must be done several segments higher than the localization of pain, to allow for the fact that fibres carrying sensations of pain and temperature enter the spinal cord and ascend for several segments before crossing the mid-line to join the lateral spinothalamic tract, and that no matter how deep the incision made at operation, the level of sensory loss always descends during the first postoperative week.

The patient is so anaesthetized during this type of operation that he can be roused when the surgeon is ready to divide the lateral spinothalamic tract. The patient co-operates by telling the surgeon the level of his sensory loss and when an adequate level is reached he is re-anaesthetized and the operation completed.

Spinothalamic cordotomies are used to relieve pain from malignant disease, especially those affecting the pelvic region. A bilateral cordotomy may be necessary for a patient who suffers from bilateral symptoms, but this procedure can produce motor weakness below the level of the surgical lesion. Bladder and bowel function are often permanently disturbed, accompanied by the loss of sexual function in the male. High cervical cordotomy may damage the respiratory pathway, innervating the diaphragm and intercostal muscles, producing an ipsilateral paralysis.

Physiotherapy treatment

Following cordotomy in the thoracic region static contractions of the back extensor muscles can begin about the seventh postoperative day, and active extension exercises when sutures are removed, approximately the tenth day.

Following a high cervical cordotomy, neck extensor muscles require retraining; static contractions can begin about the seventh postoperative day, and gentle neck mobilization when sutures are removed, approximately the tenth day. Chest care is most important if there is a diaphragmatic and intercostal muscle paralysis.

The patient should be allowed to get up between the seventh and tenth day if his general condition is satisfactory. It is important to teach him how to look after the area of pain and temperature loss. A patient with a unilateral loss should be reminded to use his normal side for testing the temperature of bath water. He must look after his affected side in the manner previously described for the paraplegic patient (p. 136).

FURTHER ADVANCES

Percutaneous cordotomy is gradually replacing open procedures, while stereotaxic cordotomy is now being developed to bring greater accuracy in lesion making. Obvious advantages of percutaneous procedures are that the patient only requires a local anaesthetic, there is no longer a painful wound, so earlier mobilization is therefore possible.

If for any reason a high cervical cordotomy is contra-indicated a stereotaxic lesion can be made in a portion of the thalamic nucleus, and is often successful in relieving pain. Certain patients whose pain may not have been adequately relieved by a surgical lesion at a lower level may derive greater benefit from thalamotomy.

BIBLIOGRAPHY

Brain (Lord) and Walton, J. N. *Diseases of the Nervous System.* Oxford University Press, 7th ed. 1969.

Brock, Samuel (ed.). *Injuries of the Brain and Spinal Cord and their Coverings,* 4th ed. 1960.

Davis, L. and Davis, R. A. *Principles of Neurological Surgery.* W. B. Saunders, 1968.

Gatz, A. J. *Manter's Essentials of Clinical Neuroanatomy and Neurophysiology.* Distributed by Blackwell, 4th ed. 1970.

Jennett, W. B. *An Introduction to Neurosurgery.* Heinemann, 2nd ed. 1970.

Lockhart, R. D., Hamilton, G. F. and Fyfe, F. W. *Anatomy of the Human Body.* Faber & Faber, 2nd ed. 1965.

Warwick, R. (ed.). *Gray's Anatomy.* Longman, 35th ed. 1973.

The Ciba Collection of medical illustrations, Vol. I

Various papers by members of the unit staff.

CHAPTER 6

Diseases of the Ear, Nose and Throat

---

revised by W. M. BUSTON, MCSP, and J. E. CASH, FCSP

Many diseases of the ear, nose or throat would not benefit from physiotherapy but there are some in which physical treatment is valuable. In these conditions the aims might be:

to aid resolution in acute and chronic sinusitis;

to help to prevent chest complications in major operations on the tongue, pharynx and larynx;

to treat facial paralysis;

to help to relieve persistent vertigo and tension in otosclerosis, Ménière's disease and labyrinthitis;

to assist in resolution of chronic inflammation of the Eustachian tube;

to help to clear up persistent ear discharge following operations on the middle ear cleft in chronic suppurative otitis media.

In order to carry out purposeful treatment, some knowledge of the anatomy and physiology of the ear and nose is helpful, together with an understanding of the various diseases for which physiotherapy is ordered.

The ear consists of three parts: the outer or external ear, the middle ear, which includes the tympanic cavity, and the internal ear or labyrinth (Fig. 6/1).

The external ear

This consists of the expanded portion or auricle of cartilage and skin, and a partly cartilaginous, partly bony tube, known as the external auditory meatus. The meatus is lined by skin continuous with that covering the auricle.

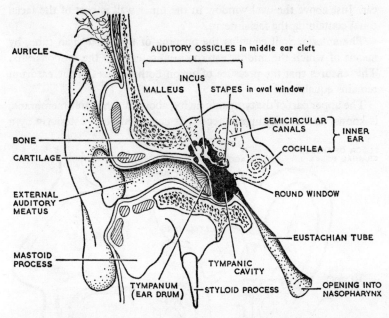

AURICLE

AUDITORY OSSICLES in middle ear cleft

INCUS

MALLEUS   STAPES in oval window

SEMICIRCULAR
CANALS

INNER
EAR

BONE

CARTILAGE

COCHLEA

EXTERNAL
AUDITORY
MEATUS

ROUND WINDOW

EUSTACHIAN TUBE

MASTOID
PROCESS

TYMPANIC
CAVITY

TYMPANUM
(EAR DRUM)   STYLOID PROCESS

OPENING INTO
NASOPHARYNX

Fig. 6/1 Diagrammatic representation of the ear showing external, middle and inner ears.

In the subcutaneous tissue of its cartilaginous portion are glands which secrete a wax. Immediately posterior to the meatus is a thin layer of bone separating the meatus from the mastoid air cells. The function of the auricle is to collect sound waves; that of the meatus is to convey the vibrations to the drumhead at the base of the tube.

The tympanic cavity

This is an air-containing space in the temporal bone, separated from the external ear by a thin semitransparent structure known as the tympanic membrane or drumhead. The inner wall is formed by the bony capsule of the internal ear. In this wall are two windows. The oval window opens into the vestibule, the central part of the internal ear. Fitted into this window, by means of a fibrous ring, is the foot-plate of the stapes. The round window, which is closed by a membrane, lies a little behind the oval window and opens into the cochlea of the inner ear. Just above the oval window in the inner wall is part of the facial canal containing the facial nerve.

The anterior wall contains the opening of the Eustachian tube, by means of which the middle ear communicates with the nasopharynx. This ensures that the pressure of air on both surfaces of the eardrum remains equal.

The upper part of the tympanic cavity, above the tympanic membrane, is known as the epitympanic recess. It communicates posteriorly by a

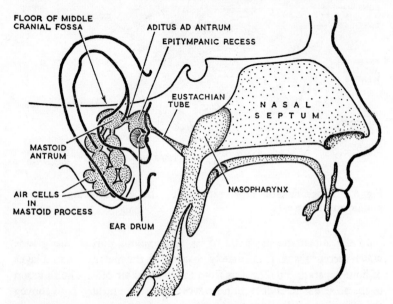

FLOOR OF MIDDLE
CRANIAL FOSSA

ADITUS AD ANTRUM

EPITYMPANIC RECESS

EUSTACHIAN
TUBE

NASAL
SEPTUM

MASTOID
ANTRUM

AIR CELLS
IN
MASTOID PROCESS

NASOPHARYNX

EAR DRUM

Fig. 6/2 The connection between throat, nose and mastoid air cells via the middle ear.

narrow passage, the aditus, with the mastoid antrum from which the mastoid air cells spread out into the surrounding bone. The whole air-containing structure, from the Eustachian tube to the mastoid air cells, is the middle ear cleft (Fig. 6/2).

Across the tympanic cavity lies a chain of tiny bones, known as the ossicles. Their purpose is to assist in the conduction of vibrations from the tympanic membrane to the inner ear. First is the malleus, resembling a hammer, attached to the tympanic membrane. It articulates with the second, the incus, resembling an anvil, and this in its turn articulates with the stapes, or stirrup, whose foot-plate fits into the oval window.

Both the walls of the tympanic cavity and the ossicles are covered with mucous membrane. This is continuous with that of the naso-pharynx, through the Eustachian tube, and with that of the mastoid antrum and air cells, through the aditus. This means that inflammation of the nasal mucous membrane can spread, by direct continuity, to the middle ear and mastoid antrum.

The internal ear or labyrinth

This lies in the petrous portion of the temporal bone. It consists of two parts: the bony labyrinth, and the membranous labyrinth. The central part of the *bony labyrinth* is the vestibule immediately deep to the tympanic cavity. The anterior part is the cochlea communicating with the vestibule. The posterior part, also communicating with the vestibule,

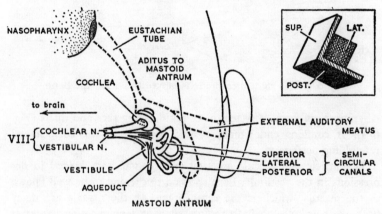

Fig. 6/3 Right bony labyrinth seen from above.

consists of three semicircular canals set at right angles to one another and representing the three planes of space. The cochlea obtains its name from its resemblance to a snail's shell. It forms a spiral tube wound round a central pillar of bone known as the modiolus. This bony tube is divided partly by bone and partly by two membranes, into an upper part, the scala vestibuli, and a lower part, the scala tympani. Each is filled with perilymph and both communicate with the middle ear, the scala vestibuli by the oval window and the scala tympani by the round window.

Into the former window is fitted the foot-plate of the stapes, and the latter is filled in by membrane. The whole labyrinth is lined with endosteum, and contains a fluid identical to cerebrospinal fluid, known as perilymph, in which floats the membranous labyrinth (Fig. 6/3).

The *membranous labyrinth* is anchored at various points to the surrounding bony labyrinth. It consists of two sacs (the utricle and saccule), three semicircular ducts and the duct of the cochlea. The semicircular ducts open at each end into the utricle; the cochlear duct opens into the saccule and the saccule and utricle communicate. The membranous

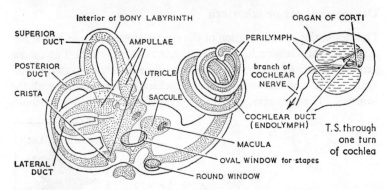

Fig. 6/4 The right membranous labyrinth within the bone.

labyrinth thus forms a system of communicating sacs and ducts (Fig. 6/4). It contains endolymph, a fluid secreted in the cochlea and resembling perilymph.

The utricle and saccule are tiny membranous sacs lodged in depressions in the vestibule. Each shows a thickening in its wall known as the macula, which is the sense organ. In the macula are many flask-like hair cells, their free edges showing long tapering processes which project into the endolymph, and come in contact with tiny crystals, the otoliths. Between the hair cells ramify the fine fibrils of the vestibular nerve.

The semicircular canals open into the utricle. One end of each canal is dilated to form the ampulla, and in each of these is found an elevation similar in structure to the macula, and known as the crista.

The cochlear duct lies between the vestibular and basilar membranes. It contains endolymph. On the basilar membrane, along the whole length of the duct, lies the organ of Corti. This consists of elongated cells with fine processes (hair cells) which are attached to a delicate membrane floating in the endolymph. The filaments of the cochlear (acoustic) nerve terminate between these cells (see Fig. 6/4).

Nervous connections of the labyrinth

The cochlear and vestibular nerves together form the eighth or auditory nerve. The former is concerned with hearing, the latter with balance.

The cells of origin of the cochlear nerve are found in the cochlear ganglion within the cochlea. Their peripheral processes terminate between the hair cells of the organ of Corti. Their central processes travel in the auditory nerve through a bony passage, the internal auditory meatus, to the pons where they relay in the cochlear nucleus. The bipolar cells of the vestibular nerve lie in the vestibular ganglion found in the internal auditory meatus. Their peripheral processes terminate between the hair cells of the cristae and maculae. Their central processes pass through the auditory nerve into the pons. Many relay in nuclei to enter the spinal cord forming the vestibulospinal tract, while others relay into the cerebellum.

Function of the labyrinth

The cochlear nerve, the cochlea and possibly the saccule too are concerned with hearing. Sound-waves set up in the ear are collected by the auricle, transmitted by the meatus and impinge on the tympanic membrane, causing it to vibrate. These vibrations are transmitted across the

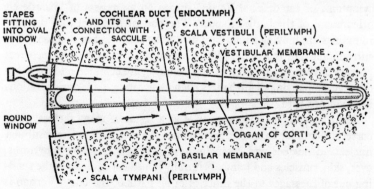

Fig. 6/5 Transmission of vibrations within the labyrinth.

tympanic cavity by the ossicles and by the air within the cavity. As the foot-plate of the stapes fits into the oval window of the vestibule, the vibrations are transmitted to the fluid in the scala vestibuli, so to the vestibular membrane, endolymph and basilar membrane (see Fig. 6/5), causing the latter to bulge into the scala tympani and so to pull on the hair cells of the organ of Corti. In this way stimuli are set up in the cochlear nerve. The round window allows for the movement of the fluid in the scala tympani.

The vestibular nerve, the semicircular ducts and the utricle are concerned with balance. When the head is moved, the fluid in the ducts and utricle tends to lag behind and consequently the hair cells of the cristae and maculae are stimulated. This results in the setting up of impulses in the filaments of the vestibular nerve. Again, the position of the head in space determines the direction of the pull of gravity on the otoliths. These pull on the tapering processes of the hair cells so that nerve impulses are generated. It is usually considered that alterations in the posture of the head influence the maculae, while movements of the head affect the cristae. Once the vestibular nerve is stimulated, appropriate messages are sent to muscles to maintain or restore balance and correct posture.

SYMPTOMS WHICH MAY ARISE IN DISEASES OF THE EAR

Pain, deafness, tinnitus (a sensation of noise caused by abnormal excitation of the auditory apparatus) and vertigo (giddiness) are common symptoms of ear defects. Vertigo means an awareness of 'disordered orientation' of the body in space. The patient may feel that the surroundings are moving round him or that he is moving in relation to his surroundings, or that some part of his body or limbs is in an incorrect posture or is unsteady. Nausea and vomiting are common and there are often accompanying disturbances such as sweating, pallor or alterations in blood pressure.

Disturbance of balance may arise as a result of many factors, since correct orientation in space depends upon the reception by the vestibular nuclei, red nucleus and cerebellum, of messages from the labyrinths, eyes, skin, muscles and joints. Naturally it also depends upon the sending out of messages to the muscles of all parts of the body. Vertigo is essentially a disorder of sensation, due to the disturbance of the vestibular end organs or the afferent pathways to the brain. We are particularly concerned here with the disturbance of the vestibular nerve and ear. In this connection, excessive accumulation of wax in the external meatus, blockage of the Eustachian tube resulting in alterations in pressure in the tympanic cavity, inflammation of the middle ear, calcification of the oval window, inflammation or intermittent action of the labyrinths, head injuries or persistent movement may all cause vertigo. It should be remembered also that giddiness may be psychogenic, and, again, that it often persists when its organic cause has been relieved. Surgery involving the labyrinth will inevitably upset the mechanism by which equilibrium and stability is maintained and vertigo may be a temporary after-effect.

The nasal cavity

This lies between the cranium and the roof of the mouth. It is divided into two halves by a median septum, cartilaginous in front and bony behind. The two halves, known as the nasal fossae, communicate with the pharynx posteriorly. Opening into each are the orifices of the various sinuses. The lateral wall of each fossa is irregular and shows three scroll-like bones, known as the turbinates. The superior and middle of these are derived from the ethmoid; the inferior is a separate bone attached to the lateral wall of the cavity. Below the turbinate bones are grooves known as the superior, middle and inferior meatus respectively.

Each nasal fossa is lined by mucous membrane. This membrane consists of an upper olfactory part, containing the bipolar cells of origin of the fibres of the olfactory nerve, and a lower respiratory part. The olfactory portion is found lining the upper one-third of the nasal septum and the lateral wall of the fossa. The respiratory portion lines the lower two-thirds of the fossa and the air sinuses. The respiratory epithelium is a specialized structure, ciliated and containing mucous glands. The submucosa contains glands, connective tissue and blood spaces which are under control of the autonomic nervous system so that the thickness of the soft tissue can be altered from time to time, thus enlarging or narrowing the air pathways.

The nose has three functions. It, together with the olfactory nerve and its central connections, is the organ of smell. It is responsible for the filtration of the air passing through it, and also for moistening and warming the air before it passes to the lungs. Should there be any nasal obstruction, these three functions may be upset.

The accessory nasal sinuses

These are air spaces in the bones of the skull, all communicating with the nasal cavity. It is usual to classify them into anterior and posterior groups. The anterior group open into the middle meatus and consist of frontal and maxillary sinuses, and anterior ethmoidal air cells. The

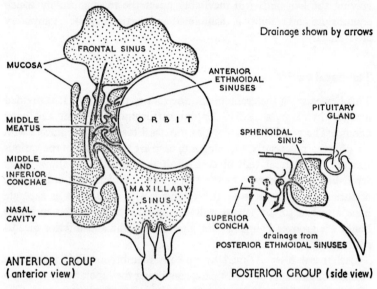

Fig. 6/6 The accessory nasal sinuses—schematic.

posterior and middle ethmoidal cells open into the superior meatus and the sphenoidal sinus into the spheno-ethmoidal recess above this. These sinuses are irregular in shape and vary in size at different ages and in different individuals. Their mucous membrane is in direct continuity with that of the nose, so that infection of the nasal mucous membrane is prone to lead to infection of that of the sinuses. The openings into the nasal cavity are small and are therefore easily blocked by swelling of the mucous membrane, and when this occurs, secretions will accumulate in the sinuses and will not be able to drain into the nose.

The maxillary sinus (Fig. 6/6) is within the maxilla. It extends from

the floor of the orbit to the roof of the mouth, and from the lateral wall
of the nasal cavity to the third molar tooth. The floor is the alveolar
process of the maxilla and is in relation to the roots of the premolar
and molar teeth. It may actually be perforated by the roots of the first
two molars.

The frontal sinus (Fig. 6/6) lies behind the superciliary arch. It
varies very much in size and shape in different individuals and is rarely
symmetrical with its fellow. In many cases it extends upwards for a
considerable distance into the frontal bone. The floor is formed by the
roof of the orbital cavity, and the sinus itself may extend laterally to the
level of the outer angle of the eye. Each sinus is separated from its
fellow by a thin plate of bone.

The ethmoidal sinuses (Fig. 6/6) consist of a group of air cells in the
lateral mass of the ethmoid. They thus lie at the upper part of the
lateral wall of the nasal cavity and in the medial wall of the orbit.

The sphenoidal sinuses (Fig. 6/6) consist of a pair of cells lying in the
body of the sphenoid behind the upper part of the nasal cavity. They
are separated from each other by a thin septum of bone.

The pharynx

The pharynx extends from the base of the skull to the level of the
cricoid cartilage and is divided into three parts. The nasopharynx
extends from the base of the skull to the soft palate and lies behind the
nasal cavity. The oropharynx extends from the soft palate to the epiglottis and lies behind the cavity of the mouth. The laryngopharynx lies
behind the larynx and extends from the epiglottis to the level of the
cricoid cartilage. The nasopharynx communicates with the nose by the
posterior nares, and with the mouth. In its lateral wall is the opening
of the Eustachian tube leading into the tympanic cavity of the ear. At
the junction of the posterior wall with the roof of this part of the
pharynx, in the mid-line, there is a large mass of lymphoid tissue known
as the pharyngeal tonsil, or adenoid, present in childhood, but tending
to disappear with age. A second mass of this tissue is found in the
oropharynx, between the pillars of the fauces on each side. This is the
oral tonsil. In both cases the function of the tissue is probably that of
protection against infection and it is for this reason that it is much more
developed in children.

ACUTE INFECTIONS OF THE MIDDLE EAR

Acute inflammation of the mucous membrane lining the middle ear cleft may follow upper respiratory tract infection or may be due to invasion through a perforated eardrum. Taylor says that one child in four in Great Britain suffers at least one attack of this condition.

There are the usual changes of inflammation together with inflammatory exudate which may be serous but can become purulent if the invading organism is virulent, the general resistance is low or treatment is not started early or is ineffective.

If the rising pressure of fluid within the middle ear is not relieved by adequate treatment the drumhead will perforate and serous or mucopurulent discharge will occur.

It is important that the condition should be recognized early or serious complications (due to the close relationship of the middle ear to other important structures) such as intracranial abscess (p. 137), meningitis (p. 186), labyrinthitis (p. 191) and mastoiditis may occur (p. 187).

The immediate treatment is to encourage drainage via the Eustachian tube, and to achieve this decongestants and steam inhalations are used. If these do not cause a rapid improvement antibiotics are started. Should the drumhead appear red and bulging a myringotomy (incision of the tympanic membrane) will probably be carried out to allow drainage and lessen the likelihood of further attacks. Any obstruction of the Eustachian tubes should later be relieved and an adenoidectomy may be advisable. If a drumhead perforation fails to heal spontaneously, a myringoplasty may be considered.

NON-SUPPURATIVE OTITIS MEDIA
(Secretory Otitis Media)

This is a condition in which chronic inflammatory changes take place in the mucosa of the middle ear. Usually a thick sticky secretion is formed. The disease occurs most commonly in young children following repeated upper respiratory tract infections. The infection may lead to thickening of the nasal mucous membrane causing obstruction of the nasopharyngeal opening of the Eustachian tube. Obstruction from enlarged tonsils may already be present.

If obstruction occurs, the air within the middle ear cleft is gradually absorbed and a negative pressure is created. This appears to cause irritation of the mucosa followed by degenerative changes, sucking out of fluid from the capillaries, and retraction of the drumhead.

The irritation of the mucous membrane and accumulation of fluid predispose towards infection, and organisms normally present in considerable numbers in the lower part of the Eustachian tube may ascend the tube.

In the course of time, as the fluid forms and its pressure rises, the drumhead will begin to bulge until it eventually perforates and a thick viscid fluid will discharge into the external auditory meatus. The condition is then sometimes known as a 'glue ear'.

The onset of this condition is not always immediately recognized, being first detected when the child is brought to the doctor suffering from catarrh, then the physician finds some degree of deafness and retraction of the drumhead.

Treatment

The object of treatment is to deal with any upper respiratory tract infection and to restore normal pressure within the middle ear cleft.

Such problems as chronic sinusitis and enlarged adenoids and tonsils are usually dealt with. Attention is paid to general health and if the ear is not discharging a myringotomy may be carried out. If the patient does not respond to this treatment, some surgeons will insert a small plastic tube (a grommet) via the eardrum into the tympanic cavity to ensure proper ventilation of the middle ear cleft. It has been found that if this is left long enough, i.e. for several months, the changes in the mucosa are improved and the ear returns to normal.

PHYSIOTHERAPY

Shortwave diathermy to the Eustachian tube has been found helpful in this condition. One method of giving this is to have the patient seated in a deck-chair with the head well supported. Medium-sized rigid electrodes are centred on either side of the face, well back and just in front of the ears. Mild heating is required and treatment starts at five to seven minutes increasing to fifteen minutes by the third treatment. Shortwave therapy is also of value in cases due to chronic infection of the nasal sinuses.

CHRONIC SUPPURATIVE OTITIS MEDIA

Ludman divides chronic suppurative otitis media into two main groups, the safe variety and the unsafe variety.

The safe variety

These include patients in whom there is chronic infection involving the mucosa but not the surrounding bone. The infection, having reached the middle ear via the Eustachian tube or a drumhead perforation, damages the mucous membrane and renders it susceptible to further infection, so that from time to time there will be bouts of mucopurulent discharge. This type of disease is usually treated conservatively by careful aural toilet and local and/or systemic antibiotics. Should hearing not improve, a hearing aid may be worn or tympanoplasty be advised.

For the persistently discharging ear via a tympanic perforation the use of shortwave therapy is often effective. Very occasionally zinc ionization may be ordered. This is applied in several ways. The principle is that bactericidal effects are obtained by the formation of a layer of zinc albuminate over the mucous membrane of the walls of the tympanic cavity. The zinc solution may reach this area through a special aural electrode, or by means of careful packing of the external auditory meatus with ribbon gauze soaked in a 2% solution of zinc sulphate. About three milliamperes may be given for ten minutes. This may be repeated weekly until the discharge ceases.

The unsafe ear

This is the case in which the bony wall of the middle ear cleft has become involved. This is so closely related to other very important structures that serious complications, even fatal to life, may occur.

Thus bone erosion may spread upwards, into the middle cranial fossa or backwards to the posterior fossa, or infection may be carried to these regions via veins passing through the petrosquamous fissure or via the mastoid veins. Such spread may be the cause of thrombosis of the superior petrosal or lateral sinuses or of intracranial abscess or/and meningitis. If the bony wall of the inner ear is involved a labyrinthitis may result, while the mastoid may become involved or the facial canal can be eroded.

The erosion of bone may be due to the chronic infection or may be the result of a cholesteatoma. A cholesteatoma is a tumour of skin cells within the ear. It is uncertain how such cells get into the middle ear, but it may be through a perforated eardrum or due to drumhead retraction resulting from negative pressure within the middle ear cleft. The epithelial cells on the centre of the normal drumhead multiply more quickly than elsewhere and, since they are not rubbed off by friction such as occurs over the rest of the body, they have the special property of migration, moving outwards on the drumhead and along the external auditory meatus. This cannot occur if they become enclosed within the middle ear and so they form a gradually increasing collection of cells which often becomes infected so that a type of skin cyst develops. As this grows it tends to erode bone and may intrude into the facial canal, mastoid air cells, labyrinth and intracranial fossae.

Patients with 'unsafe ears' usually suffer from tinnitus, earache, diminished hearing and ear discharge. If headache and vertigo develop they may well be a warning of invasion of the cranial fossae. Facial palsy will indicate erosion of the facial canal.

Mastoid operations are nearly always necessary for these patients because of the serious complications. There are different operations but they all aim at forming one large clean cavity, lined by skin and communicating with the external auditory meatus. All diseased tissue and cholesteatoma processes are removed, as may be the malleus and incus.

These patients usually have the sutures removed at about five days and may then be allowed to go home, but the ear will continue to discharge until the skin lining is properly formed and this sometimes takes a very long time.

PHYSIOTHERAPY

Shortwave diathermy is sometimes ordered if the ear discharge persists and it is often successful in helping to clear up the discharge.

Should facial palsy occur treatment will be necessary (p. 191).

OTOSCLEROSIS

This condition attacks the bony capsule of the labyrinths. It is characterized by a localized absorption of the bone and replacement by a thick woven bone. The cause is unknown. It usually first appears between the ages of 15 and 45 and produces varying degrees of deafness according to the site of the bony change.

The disease is particularly liable to involve the annular ring and foot-plate of the stapes and may spread to the oval window. The stapes thus becomes fixed and can no longer respond to sound-waves so that conductive deafness results.

Sometimes the cochlear labyrinth is involved and there may also be compression of the structures at the internal auditory meatus. Involvement of the vestibular labyrinth may result in vertigo. Thus deafness may not be the only problem.

Treatment

Conservative treatment will include the wearing of a hearing aid, and when hearing loss is progressing the patient should be taught to lip-read.

For suitable patients in whom the stapes is becoming fixed, a stapedectomy is often very successful.

In this operation the greater part of the stapes is removed through a permeatal incision. A hole is drilled in the foot-plate, which has been left in situ, and a small plastic piston covered by a vein graft is attached to the incus and its other end is fitted through the hole in the foot-plate. The ear is packed with narrow ribbon gauze for a few days and then a cotton wool pack is substituted for about two weeks.

Immediately after the operation the patient is nursed in side lying on the unaffected side, but is usually allowed up next day and goes home on the third to fifth day. For a few days head movements may make the patient feel giddy, but this is usually controlled by drugs.

PHYSIOTHERAPY

Occasionally vertigo persists and physiotherapy may then be ordered. The giddiness is aggravated by any change of position and is particularly bad on sudden movements of the head or eyes. For this reason the patient tends to hold the head and eyes still and to move the trunk slowly and carefully. The neck and shoulder muscles therefore become tense and often remain so, long after the giddiness has permanently disappeared.

The object of physical treatment is to gain relaxation of tense muscles and to overcome the fear of giddiness, until it completely ceases and the patient is capable of carrying out normal activities with normal self-confidence. If these aims are not achieved, the tenseness continues and activities are limited through fear of the unpleasant sensation of vertigo. The exact routine of exercise varies. It is common to begin with eye movements, first slowly, then quickly, and then a combination of both. The use of long and short focus is also valuable. Provided that the head is supported, head bending forward and rotation may also be given. Head backward bending is often avoided as it seems to produce more vertigo. On the next day, the same movements may be practised in the long-sitting position and head rolling and head extension may be added, performed first with the eyes open and then with eyes closed. These movements should also be performed slowly at first and then quickly, and then changing rapidly from one speed to another. Shoulder movements to gain relaxation are now added and slow trunk movements. The patient can then join a class of other patients, so that the spirit of competition may enter into the treatment. Exercises in sitting, stressing trunk and head flexion and extension, are given, and standing, trying to gain steady balance, is added. Progression is made daily by adding exercises in standing and by using changes of posture, first with the eyes open and then closed. Ball throwing makes a useful exercise to obtain balance and co-ordination. Ball work may be developed in standing and walking so that moving about freely is encouraged. Later balance walking, walking round objects and passing other people should all be used.

Patients vary in their progress and exercises must be chosen accordingly. The mental make-up of the patient has a great deal to do with the rate of recovery. The treatment should be pressed to the limit of tolerance of the individual, and encouragement given in order to restore confidence. The patient has to learn that a movement which makes him a little giddy has no untoward effects, and the next day that same movement may well fail to produce giddiness.

MÉNIÈRE'S DISEASE

This is a disease first described by Prosper Ménière in 1861, in which there is an increase in the quantity of endolymph in the labyrinths. It is characterized by sudden attacks of vertigo, nausea and vomiting, tinnitus and deafness. The attack may last less than an hour, several hours or longer and there may be premonitory signs such as a dull ache in the ear or there may be no warning. Some patients have a history of tinnitus and increasing deafness in one or both ears, but otherwise the ears are normal.

The actual cause is unknown though many theories exist. One fairly widely accepted theory is that there is spasm of the blood vessels supplying the labyrinth, resulting in ischaemia. This theory is reinforced by the fact that vasodilator drugs and cervical sympathectomy appear to bring about an improvement in the condition. It is also found that attacks are sometimes precipitated by stress and anxiety and exposure to cold.

The attacks are slightly more common in men than women and first occur before the age of 50.

Once an attack has occurred the patient tends to become tense and depressed. This is partly due to the tinnitus and partly because the patient is frightened of how this condition may affect his everyday life. An attack may be so severe that the patient may fall and be quite unable to walk and such an attack might be serious in his work or, for example, when driving a car. The vertigo may not be as severe or prolonged as this and after one or two attacks the condition may never occur again. Attacks can usually be controlled by conservative treatment.

Medical treatment

This is directed towards the reduction of the hypertension of endolymph, relief of fear and depression, and control of symptoms. During a severe attack the patient should lie flat in bed with the head supported by pillows. The nausea is controlled by drugs such as Stemetil (prochlorperazine maleate), and sedatives and tranquillizers will relieve anxiety. Between attacks salt and water restriction and vasodilator drugs such as nicotinic acid and Priscol (tolazoline hydrochloride) are often valuable.

If this treatment does not prove effective, conservative surgical treatment or radical surgery in the form of total destruction of the labyrinth may prove necessary.

Surgical treatment

This may be *conservative*—in the form of surgical sympathectomy, decompression of the labyrinth or selective destruction of the labyrinth by placing the tip of an ultrasound applicator on one end of the lateral semicircular canal.

Ménière's disease may also be treated by *total destruction of a labyrinth*—by withdrawing the membranous lateral semicircular duct through an opening in the bony capsule or by removing the utricle through the oval window.

These operations are followed by vertigo, particularly severe after total destruction, but usually gradually lessening over a period of several weeks. When there has been selective destruction the patient is warned that he may suffer from mild attacks of vertigo for about three months. During this time vertigo is controlled by drugs but physiotherapy is often helpful.

PHYSIOTHERAPY

This is ordered to help the patient to overcome persistent vertigo (p. 188).

LABYRINTHITIS

This condition occurs as a result of the spread of infection from a chronic suppurative otitis media (p. 186). It tends to involve both vestibular and cochlear parts of the labyrinth and is therefore characterized by hearing loss and disturbance of balance. There may be acute attacks of vertigo, when the patient falls and vomits. When walking he tends to use a broad base and falls towards the side of the affected ear.

The treatment is primarily directed towards the chronic otitis media and consists of an intensive course of antibiotics. If the attacks do not clear, total destruction of the labyrinth usually gives full recovery in four to six weeks.

Should any vertigo persist, physiotherapy may be ordered (p. 188).

FACIAL PALSY

Facial palsy is one of the complications of disease of the middle and inner ear. The facial nerve can be compressed or damaged in any part of its course, but as a complication of aural disease it is in its intratemporal course that it will be affected. During this part of the course the nerve, in the narrow bony facial canal, runs from the internal auditory meatus laterally above the labyrinth for a short distance. It makes a right-angled turn back (the genu) then runs down and back in the medial wall of the tympanic cavity (Fig. 6/7) and finally passes vertically down in the posterior wall of the cavity surrounded by mastoid air cells. The bony wall of the canal is very thin and it may actually be deficient at one or more points.

Due to its position the canal and nerve may readily be involved in ear diseases and in surgery, the nerve becoming inflamed, compressed or injured.

Acute infections of the middle ear can involve the sheath of the nerve,

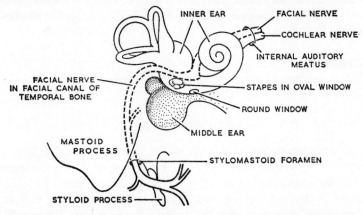

Fig. 6/7 Lateral view of the intratemporal course of the right facial nerve.

especially if an infected mastoid air cell lies just above the nerve in the absence of the bony wall of the canal.

Erosion of the bony wall of the canal is liable to occur in chronic suppurative otitis media, either by infection or a cholesteatoma.

In surgery the nerve may be damaged during the operation or by the displacement of fragments of bone. It may be compressed by haemorrhage or oedema.

In addition to involvement in diseases of the ear the nerve may also be damaged in this part of its course in fractures of the temporal bone. Idiopathic facial palsy (Bell's palsy) can also occur. The cause is unknown and there is no apparent disease of the ear. One theory (Groves) is that vasospasm results in swelling and ischaemia and consequently compression of the nerve. Such ischaemia could be the result of exposure to draughts and cold.

Types of lesion

The lesion may be a neurapraxia due either to compression by blood or exudate, or caused by bruising. Alternatively, there may be degeneration of the nerve if compression is not relieved or the nerve is damaged during surgery. A combination of both types of lesion is possible.

Treatment

A very careful assessment has to be made before treatment can be decided upon, in order to estimate the type and level of the lesion. Such assessment includes a test of motor function, nerve conductivity tests and strength-duration measurements, electromyography, and lacrimation, hearing and taste tests. Treatment is then decided upon according to the above tests and the speed of onset and progression of the paralysis.

Facial paralysis developing during acute middle ear infections will usually recover completely without special treatment when the primary condition is dealt with (p. 191).

Should the paralysis occur in chronic suppurative otitis media, exploration is usually considered essential. The facial canal is opened and if there is fibrosis and degeneration, the sheath of the nerve is incised, fibrous tissue removed and a nerve graft carried out. Any cutaneous nerve may be used. Recovery is likely to be slow—some months—and may not be complete.

The onset of facial palsy immediately after aural surgery is likely to indicate that the nerve has been damaged. The surgeon will explore at once and carry out a decompression or graft according to what he finds.

A delayed paralysis following surgery will indicate either too tight packing in the ear, slight contusion of the nerve or, if the paralysis is increasing, bleeding into the facial canal. This will require either removal of the packing or exploration of the facial canal.

Idiopathic facial palsy rarely requires surgical treatment. Many patients recover within two to three weeks without treatment. Some patients recover very slowly, those in whom some nerve fibres have degenerated. A few never get full recovery and in these there has been total degeneration. Some surgeons treat the patient with A.C.T.H. and claim excellent results, others have tried decompression but as yet there is no certain proof that this is effective. Usually treatment is medical and includes reassurance of the patient, care of the eye, exercises for the facial muscles and support for the paralysed muscles.

In all cases general care of the patient as described above for idiopathic facial palsy is essential and physiotherapy is usually ordered.

Physiotherapy

Physiotherapy is usually ordered whatever the type of lesion, since there will be a short or long period before full recovery of the facial muscles. In some cases complete recovery may not occur.

The measures which may be taken include: nerve conductivity tests; strength-duration curves; movement using proprioceptive neuromuscular facilitation (P.N.F.) techniques; infra-red therapy; occasionally ice therapy; occasionally electrical stimulation.

NERVE CONDUCTIVITY TESTS

When facial palsy appears immediately after surgery, a nerve conductivity test may be requested at an early stage, from three to ten days. If the nerve has been completely severed there will be immediate failure in conductivity and no muscle response, whereas if there is a muscle twitch the nerve cannot have been severed.

The usual method of carrying out the test is to have the patient in the lying position. A small button electrode is placed at the exit of the nerve from the stylomastoid foramen and the indifferent electrode on the neck. A pulse of one millisecond is used. The intensity of current needed to obtain a minimal visible contraction on the normal side is compared with that needed on the affected side.

STRENGTH-DURATION CURVES

These are carried out, when necessary, to determine the type of nerve lesion and the patient's progress.

MOVEMENTS

While there is no ability to contract the muscles the physiotherapist may do the movement for the patient, who is asked to try to 'feel' it and to attempt to hold it. As power begins to return the patient tries to join in and proprioceptive neuromuscular facilitation (P.N.F.) techniques may be used. A spatula can be placed inside the cheek and the patient is asked to pull the cheek in as it is pressed out by the spatula.

INFRA-RED AND ICE THERAPY

The small, delicate facial muscles waste quickly, and can become fibrotic and contracted if recovery is delayed. Stimulation of the circulation and nutrition is therefore valuable, consequently gentle heat is often given before movement. Ice could be used but it has the disadvantage of causing rupture of tiny superficial veins, which is not desirable on the face.

ELECTRICAL STIMULATION

This is rarely used today but occasionally if a patient cannot get the 'idea' of the movement, when paralysis has been present for some time, electrical stimulation can be used until he has acquired the 'feel' and knows what to try to do.

In some patients as the nerve recovers, associated movements tend to occur, for example, as the patient closes the eye the corner of the mouth shoots up. It may be difficult to prevent this but if the patient is shown what is happening he can be encouraged to make an effort to control it.

The physiotherapist will encourage the patient to take care of the eye, stressing that he should not go out without covering it. If trouble does occur she must report it at once.

CHRONIC RHINITIS

Chronic inflammation of the mucous lining of the nose is characterized by nasal obstruction and rhinorrhoea, sometimes accompanied by bouts of sneezing. It may be allergic in origin or due to vasomotor instability.

In allergic rhinitis the cause is often an inhaled or ingested allergen such as in house dust or in particular foods. The patients are treated by avoidance of the allergen, if it can be discovered, or by hyposensitization, antihistamines and sometimes one long-lasting injection of methylprednisolone acetate. Very occasionally a course of zinc ionization is ordered. It is possible that this may reduce the sensitivity of the mucous membrane. The first treatment is usually given for five minutes and six milliamperes should be tolerated. Three treatments are given and the time is progressed from five to seven and then to ten minutes.

The course often proves successful in relieving the condition for a period of several months. It should be given (in this country) in April or May and can be repeated after three or four months if necessary. In carrying out the treatment, care is necessary not to produce a haemorrhage, and very careful packing of the nasal cavities is required. This packing should be done in the Ear, Nose and Throat department. This treatment is not often used today.

When the cause is vasomotor instability, the probable explanation lies in a lack of balance between the parasympathetic and sympathetic innervation of the nasal mucous membrane. Normally the balance is only disturbed temporarily by such factors as smoke, extremes of temperature, etc., but in some individuals there seems to be a permanent upset in favour of parasympathetic stimulation resulting in persistent vasodilatation and increased mucus secretion. Eventually the mucous membrane becomes hypertrophied and causes nasal obstruction, often worse at night, disturbing sleep. The cause of this instability is unknown but factors such as extremes of temperature and humidity, hormonal imbalance, anxiety, anger or excitement appear to precipitate an attack.

In some the nasal obstruction is most marked while in others the excessive watery discharge causes the patient to complain of a persistent 'runny' nose. When nasal obstruction is present, shortwave or microwave therapy often prove very successful and very occasionally zinc ionization is ordered.

Shortwave therapy. Shortwave therapy is given two or three times weekly for six weeks. One method is to use medium-sized, rigid electrodes positioned over the maxillary antra and treatment is given, progressing from seven to fifteen minutes. Some physiotherapists use the cross-fire technique, giving shortwave treatment to the antra for five to ten minutes each way.

Zinc ionization is applied in the same way as for allergic rhinitis.

NASAL SINUSITIS

This is an inflammation of the mucous membrane lining the nasal sinuses. It may be acute or chronic. The maxillary sinus is most often affected, but all the sinuses on one side can be involved or all the sinuses of both sides (pansinusitis).

Acute sinusitis

Acute sinusitis is most often caused by the virus of the common cold. It also results from chronic dental infection, trauma or infected tonsils and/or adenoids. Infection is especially likely to occur if there is partial obstruction of the opening from the nose to the sinus, such as may be present when there is a deflected nasal septum, enlarged adenoids or an allergic state of the nose causing swelling of the nasal mucous membrane. Sinusitis is also often associated with chest infections.

The inflammation is characterized by swelling and exudate with increased secretion of mucus. If the organism is virulent, the patient's resistance low or the exudate cannot drain adequately, due to blockage of the opening, the exudate may become purulent.

Symptoms are general and local. There is a slight rise in temperature, a feeling of general malaise and headache. Pain is usually present, sometimes with tenderness on pressure. If the maxillary sinus is affected pain is felt in the cheek in the region of the upper teeth; in frontal sinusitis it is just under the upper margin of the orbital cavity; in ethmoidal sinusitis at the upper part of the side of the nose.

Nasal discharge is mucoid at first in most patients, but after a few days may become purulent. Once adequate drainage is established, relief of pain may be expected and within a few days the condition may be cleared and discharge ceases.

TREATMENT

For patients who suffer from sinusitis, prophylactic treatment is valuable. Measures which improve general health are important. Plenty of fresh air, sunlight and a good mixed diet are ordered. The patient is warned not to fly or swim if he has a cold, and diving and jumping into the water are best avoided.

During an attack treatment is directed towards obtaining drainage. Inhalations and ephedrine nasal drops will help to decongest the mucous membrane. Pain is relieved by sedatives and infection controlled by systemic antibiotics. Occasionally shortwave therapy is ordered, but it must be given with great care if drainage is not yet established. Its purpose is to stimulate the circulation and vitality of the mucous membrane without increasing tissue metabolism or the activity of the micro-organisms. For this reason very mild doses are given. The electrodes should be arranged so that all the walls of the affected sinus are treated.

When drainage commences, shortwave therapy is more effective since there is less danger of increasing congestion and pain. Stronger, thermal doses are now suitable. These should be repeated several times daily. As discharge decreases, treatments need not be so frequent.

If the condition does not clear with this treatment the surgeon may decide to clear the exudate by antral washouts. A puncture is made through the inferior meatus and normal saline is injected into the antrum. The fluid and exudate will return via the normal opening into the nose. Several washouts may be necessary and shortwave should be continued until the sinus is clear.

Chronic sinusitis

Chronic sinusitis often develops insidiously following either an acute attack which fails to resolve completely, or repeated colds or tooth infection. Permanent changes take place in the lining membrane of the sinus and sometimes in the bony walls. The mucous membrane becomes thickened and fibrotic, cilia disappear, mucous glands hypertrophy and a thick sticky mucus is difficult to move. The secretions therefore stagnate and become infected.

Constant absorption of toxins and swallowing of infected material upsets the general health and causes chronic gastritis so that the patient is likely to complain of headache, tiredness and digestive disturbances.

Local symptoms are mucopurulent nasal discharge and pain in the face, worse in the morning since secretions have accumulated during the night. A postnasal drip is often very worrying to the patient.

Treatment may be medical, minor surgery or radical surgery. Physiotherapy is often ordered.

MEDICAL TREATMENT
This will include the relief of symptoms. Nasal decongestants and ephedrine drops will relieve the nasal obstruction and analgesics will reduce the headache.

Infection will be controlled by antibiotics.

Any allergic factor may be dealt with by antihistamines.

Accumulated secretions can be removed by antral lavage or, if necessary, by intranasal antrostomy (the making of an additional opening between sinus and nasal cavity).

The condition of the mucous membrane will be improved by short-wave therapy.

SURGERY

Minor surgical measures may be necessary for the removal of any factors contributing to the chronic condition such as tooth infection, nasal polyps or a deflected nasal septum.

Radical surgery is used if other measures are not successful. The aim is to clear the cavity either by removing the mucous lining or, as in the case of the ethmoidal air cells, by breaking down the walls of these cells and converting them into one clean cavity. A permanent opening is made from the sinus to the nasal cavity.

One widely accepted procedure for a chronic maxillary sinusitis is the Caldwell-Luc operation. In this the sinus is approached through an incision in the mouth just below the gingivolabial fold. The mucous lining of the antrum is removed and a permanent opening formed low in the lateral wall of the nasal cavity. The operation is followed by inhalations, nose-drops and mouthwashes and the patient is warned not to blow his nose or wear his dentures until the wound is healed. Some surgeons follow the operation by antral lavages. The patient usually gets up the day after the operation and is allowed to go home when antral washouts are clear, in about seven days.

PHYSIOTHERAPY

Physiotherapy is often ordered as part of either the medical or surgical treatment. Heat by shortwave diathermy will increase the circulation and so aid the nutrition of the mucous membrane and the resolution of the chronic inflammatory condition.

Pre- and postoperative breathing exercises are most important. Many cases of chronic sinusitis already have a chest condition, often asthma or bronchiectasis. Thus before radical surgery, as in the Caldwell-Luc operation, the patient is taught coughing, general and localized breathing and told about the positions which may be used postoperatively.

As soon as possible after the operation the patient will be nursed propped up, and breathing exercises are given in this position. Tipping is not given unless especially ordered by the surgeon since there is always the danger of the secretions from the chest passing into the sinus and causing further infection and, in addition, the head-down position is very uncomfortable, there is severe headache and the antrum feels 'as if it will burst'. If it is necessary because of chest complications, the patient may lie flat and roll from side to side but the head-down position should be avoided.

EPISTAXIS

The physiotherapist does not treat the condition of persistent or recurrent nose-bleeding, but it can occur when physical treatment is being given. Consequently she should know under what circumstances bleeding is likely and what to do in the event of its occurrence. Some of the possible conditions are:

acute inflammation of the nasal or sinus mucous membrane. Bleeding is caused by the congestion of the blood vessels and is often precipitated by nose blowing;

in hay fever for the same reason as above;

in the presence of dilated vessels on the antero-inferior part of the nasal septum;

in patients suffering from high blood pressure and atheroma;

in anaemia when there may be a deficiency of thromboplastin and blood platelets;

following surgery;

following injury to the nose and face.

Normally a nose-bleed arrests spontaneously within a very short time, but if it persists the patient should sit, leaning forward over a bowl, and the lower half of the nose should be pinched between the thumb and fingers. The face may be bathed with a cold sponge or cloth. Should the bleeding continue for long a doctor should be called. The nose may then be packed or ruptured vessels cauterized.

If bleeding is not successfully controlled the patient will probably be admitted to hospital so that the nose can be packed, blood loss made up by blood transfusion and the general condition checked for possible cause and treatment for such conditions as hypertension, anaemia or nasal or sinus malignant growths, instituted.

MALIGNANT DISEASE OF THE LARYNX AND PHARYNX

Treatment of malignant disease of these areas will be by cytotoxic drugs, radiotherapy, surgery or a combination of all three. When surgery is undertaken pre- and postoperative physiotherapy is necessary.

Various operations are carried out. These may involve a partial laryngectomy through a vertical mid-line incision; a total laryngectomy, or a pharyngolaryngectomy, sometimes involving part of the oesophagus. In some cases a block dissection of the cervical lymph nodes is also necessary. The incision commonly used in the latter cases consists of two curved transverse incisions, one at the level of the hyoid bone and

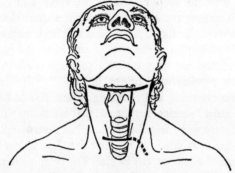

Fig. 6/8 Incisions for total laryngectomy and pharyngolaryngectomy.

the other at the level of the first or second ring of the trachea, and a vertical incision one inch (2.5 cm) from mid-line (Fig. 6/8). Drainage tubes are often used when a block dissection is done.

The pharynx may be reconstructed by skin flaps from the neck, a Teflon graft or by abdominal organs, for example, the 'pulling up' of stomach or transplantation of colon and suturing to the pharynx. If the oesophagus is involved, abdominal organ reconstruction is the method chosen in order to preserve peristalsis. In this case there will be an additional abdominal incision and a greater possibility of chest complications. In total laryngectomy and laryngopharyngectomy there will be a permanent tracheostomy and the natural voice will be lost, but the patient can be trained to use an oesophageal voice.

Whatever operative procedure is chosen, haemorrhage and chest complications are possible postoperative problems. There is danger of inhalation of blood, and inability to cough up blood and mucus may lead to infection and partial lung collapse. Patients are usually, therefore, in the Intensive Care Unit for the first 24 to 48 hours. As soon as possible they are propped up into the half-lying position. The head and neck, in the more severe operations, are carefully supported by extensive dressings and bandages and pillows. Usually the patient starts to sit out of bed the day after the operation—the length of time being increased each day—and will probably go home at about the end of three weeks.

PHYSIOTHERAPY

Pre-operative training in breathing and coughing is essential. The patient must learn to use all parts of the lungs and how to cough effectively. To achieve the latter he is taught a short sharp expiration sometimes known as 'huffing'. Arm, head and neck movements should be checked. It is helpful if the patient can meet the physiotherapist before the operation and so gain reassurance and confidence.

Postoperative physiotherapy begins in the intensive care unit and concentrates on breathing and coughing. These should be timed to fit in with the regular 'sucking out' periods. If necessary tipping may be used for laryngectomy patients but if there has been oesophageal reconstruction tipping is avoided for the first few days unless there is lung collapse, though the patient can lie flat. For these patients percussion must be given with great care; often only vibrations are used. The vital treatment is frequent breathing exercises and coughing.

When moving patients with these extensive incisions and drainage tubes in situ, great care must be taken to support the head. Any extension of the neck should be avoided because of the strain on the pharyngeal stitches which would result. The patient is very apprehensive of moving the head and neck, and gentle movements may be necessary later when the surgeon permits, though they usually recover naturally by the time the patient goes home.

When block dissection of cervical lymph nodes has been carried out there will be considerable cutting of muscles and other soft tissues and movement of the shoulder may be painful and limited. This must be watched for and if necessary shoulder exercises are started four to five days after the operation and progressed during the next two to three weeks.

REFERENCES AND BIBLIOGRAPHY

Best, C. H. and Taylor, N. B. *The Living Body*. Chapman & Hall Ltd, 4th ed. 1959.

Ludman, H. *Diseases of the Ear, Nose and Throat*. Pitman Medical and Scientific Publishing Co., 1969.

Ballantyne, J. and Groves, J. (eds.). *Scott Brown's Diseases of the Ear, Nose and Throat*. Butterworth, 3rd ed. 1971. Vol. 1 Basic Sciences, Vol. 2 The Ear, Vol. 3 The Nose, Vol. 4 The Throat.

Groves, J. 'Facial Paralysis'. Vol. 2 *ibid*.

Taylor, L. 'Acute Inflammation of Middle Ear'. Vol. 2 *ibid*.

CHAPTER 7

Injuries to Soft Tissues—I

by M. K. PATRICK, OBE, MCSP, SRP

Whilst the ensuing chapter deals with trauma and its effects on soft tissues, it must be remembered that these tissues can show inflammatory changes as a result of other pathological causes. These conditions are discussed in other chapters.

The principle of treatment for all will be to establish the cause of the tissue abnormality and then to deal with it.

The aims of local treatment are: prevention of further tissue damage; reduction of effusion; prevention of loss of range of movement; prevention of muscle atrophy; regaining full power and function; and restoration of confidence in the affected part or limb.

PHYSICAL EXAMINATIONS

When a patient presents himself after an injury with a shoulder pain, knee pain or back pain it is essential to determine which structures have been damaged and to what degree. The treatment will be based on these findings.

The history of the injury that the patient gives will reveal the time of the incident and how it occurred. The physical signs and symptoms indicate the results of the mechanical failure. It is by understanding these that the tissue damage can be determined. It is obvious that if a knee is found to have spasm of the hamstring group of muscles and atonia of the quadriceps, with local spasm around a large haematoma of the thigh, that the latter is the site of the lesion. However, when large 'joints' are involved the massive reaction to injury can make it difficult to decide exactly which tissues are damaged.

The tests are made by a doctor initially, but it is important that the physiotherapist should understand them and be able to repeat them if necessary. Some of the physical tests that are carried out are actually diagnostic, but most of them are indications. When they are 'positive' together with physical signs, a gradual picture is built up. Other tests will be tried and found not to be positive and so the field of diagnosis is narrowed until either a definite lesion can be pinpointed, or a general diagnosis made. It is important for the physiotherapist to understand the significance of these tests. Whilst the total tests are legion the most common ones are discussed here with the examination of the area.

EXAMINATION OF THE SHOULDER

A shoulder cannot be examined for a lesion, in isolation. It is essential to consider the shoulder girdle and whole upper limb as well, since they are all functionally interrelated, and any impairment of the action of one part often disturbs the harmony of movement of the whole region. The cervical spine must also be examined, as some muscles acting on and influencing the shoulder region take their attachment from the cervical spine. The nerve roots of the cervical and brachial plexi provide the myotomes and dermatomes to the arm and shoulder region.

History

It is often better to obtain the history before the patient is asked to undress, then the clinical picture that the examiner is forming from the history can be checked against the observation of the patient as he undresses.

Attention should be paid to the onset of symptoms, method of injury, the forces involved and the signs and symptoms that the patient has observed. Previous injuries, painful episodes or loss of movement should also be noted. Patients do not always readily associate their previous pain as being relevant. The large range of the shoulder joint and girdle movement makes it particularly vulnerable to the effects of wear and tear, and it is not uncommon to find that the middle-aged and elderly have some limitation of range. A woman may admit that she has been unable to raise her arm to do her hair, or a man may say he has pain when carrying a heavy weight. Any previous treatment they may have had, and their response to it, may be significant; as may the nature of their work and hobbies over the years.

Observation

Observation should begin as soon as the patient arrives. The patient's general posture should be noted. Some patients will hold the arm close to the body and support its weight at the elbow with the other hand. This is usually a sign that the patient is in great pain.

When the patient undresses it is important to watch not only the movements but the expression on the patient's face to verify his reaction to any pain that may have been experienced. The actual removal of clothes normally involves rotation of the shoulder joint and girdle, as well as a rhythmical sequence of movement which is particular to the person. Any pain or limitation of range in the region can interrupt this sequence and it becomes laboured. If, however, undressing is relatively easy, it is possible that the lesion is of nerve root origin rather than in the shoulder region, since it is the traction strain of the weight of the arm on the nerve root which causes the pain.

Once the patient is suitably undressed he should be observed in the relaxed standing position. The posture of the head, neck and shoulder girdle and the contours of the areas are compared for any deviation from the normal. An elevated shoulder may be associated with an increase in muscle tension due to pain, but it could be the result of changes which have developed over the years as a result of occupational habit. The rest of the examination is conducted with the patient sitting.

Atrophy is most readily observed in muscles such as the lateral rotators of the shoulder, and either part or the whole of deltoid. Judgement has to be based on comparison with the unaffected side. Gross alteration of contour such as occurs with dislocation or displaced fractures is readily seen. Swelling is unusual in the shoulder region as the capsule is loose and can accommodate any increase in synovial fluid that may occur.

Following a direct injury a localized haematoma may be observed, but bruising from damaged blood vessels at a deeper level may be considerably delayed. This is because the deeper structures are tightly compressed by overlying muscles, and the blood and other exudate tracks downwards through the relatively loose fascia to appear distal to the site of the injury.

Palpation

This must be carried out gently and carefully to ensure that the patient remains as relaxed as possible. A sound understanding of normal anatomy and considerable experience is needed, before a precise interpretation of the findings of palpation can be made. A generalized palpation is carried out to ascertain the temperature of the area, the mobility and elasticity of the skin, the degree of muscle tone and area of maximum tenderness.

Specific palpations, in association with particular movements, are then undertaken to localize the pain and tissue structure involved if muscle relaxation can be obtained.

ACUTE JOINT INFLAMMATION

The examiner compresses the shoulder between flat hands placed on the anterior and posterior aspects of the shoulder joint area. An increase of pain will be experienced by the patient if there is an acute inflammatory state, when tension is increased within the joint.

BICIPITAL TENDONITIS

When the shoulder muscles are relaxed the intertubercular sulcus (bicipital groove) can be palpated. Localized tenderness is found. This is made worse when the patient is asked to supinate his forearm and flex his elbow against resistance.

SUBACROMIAL (SUBDELTOID) BURSITIS

Deep palpation just lateral to the lateral border of the acromion process of the scapula will elicit tenderness in the subacromial bursa if it is inflamed. This bursa is susceptible to trauma due to its position under the subacromial arch. Passive compression of the bursa can also be carried out by placing one hand under the flexed elbow and the other over the acromion process. The humerus is moved passively upwards, thus compressing the bursa, and this causes acute pain if the bursa is swollen.

SUPRASPINATUS TENDONITIS

This tendon can be palpated when the arm is adducted and rotated medially, thus bringing its area of attachment on the upper margin of the greater tuberosity out from under cover of the acromial arch. The examiner then places a finger transversely across the tendon and pain is elicited if there is tendonitis present.

JOINT LINE PALPATION

This can be palpated anteriorly and posteriorly, but only if the muscles are fully relaxed. In the elderly, whose muscle tone is less, it is often possible to elicit joint line tenderness which is very specific and localized, indicating chronic osteoarthrosis.

ACUTE CAPSULITIS

The region of tenderness is much larger than that in the chronic osteoarthrotic patient. If the arm is moved passively in a lateral direction, with some traction on the humerus, an increase of pain will be felt by the patient with an acute lesion of the capsule.

STERNOCLAVICULAR AND ACROMIOCLAVICULAR LESIONS

These joints may show a slight swelling and feel warm on palpation if there is an acute traumatic lesion of either joint. They are 'sprung' by finger pressure being applied to the bone (near the joint) to cause movement at the joint and so movement of the damaged soft tissues. Each joint can be 'sprung' by placing the fingers over the appropriate end of the clavicle and depressing it. This stress on the soft tissues of the joint causes acute pain if damage is present.

NERVE ROOT IRRITATION

The pain from this type of lesion follows the dermatome of the nerve root, and it may only be apparent at certain points. A fifth cervical nerve root irritation nearly always produces an area of acute tenderness at the insertion of deltoid. A similar tender area can be palpated just above the superior angle of the scapula. If it is thought that the lesion is of cervical origin, then the usual tests for root pain should be carried out, e.g. does nerve stretching cause pain.

Movement

From the history, observation and palpation, the examiner will have built up a picture of the lesion that he thinks has occurred. It only remains to test the appropriate movements to conclude the examination. Since pain and its resulting muscle spasm are so often such paramount features of shoulder lesions it is advisable to carry out all movements on the unaffected side first. Then the patient is likely to co-operate better in demonstrating similar movements on the affected side. All of these movements must be carefully recorded for comparison of one shoulder with the other, and at a later stage to assess progress. The point at which pain is experienced should also be carefully noted. When the patient is asked to raise his arm, he should be observed from the rear and the examiner's thumb placed on the inferior angle of the scapula, the forefinger on the posterior rim of the glenoid cavity, the other fingers on the arm. Movement of the arm, and the point in movement at which the scapula moves, can be felt. Resisted movements will be tested to ascertain if there is any muscle weakness. Again the unaffected side is tested first and used as the comparison.

Passive movements of the injured shoulder are often not possible because of the acute pain and muscle spasm which is present. Usually if a passive movement can be made without causing pain, whereas a similar movement performed actively causes pain, it is reasonable to assume that the muscle, or the structures being compressed by the muscular contraction, are damaged. In the shoulder region this is not altogether true. If a pain-free passive movement can be performed it is usually a sign that the lesion is not in the shoulder region, but is that of a nerve root irritation, since in shoulder lesions there is usually too much muscle spasm to allow a passive movement of any great range to be performed.

Painful arc syndrome

This is the name often given to describe an injury to the rotator cuff. When the patient is asked to raise his arm above his head, the first 50° to 70° of movement are usually pain-free. When attempting further movement the patient may be seen to elevate his shoulder instead of producing pure abduction (reversed scapulohumeral rhythm, see Fig. 7/1, p. 210). If the patient persists with the movement the pain usually fades after about 30° to 40° of the painful arc. This pain is caused by a lesion of the rotator cuff muscles (infra- and supraspinatus, subscapularis and teres minor) at their point of attachment to the capsule, which is compressed under the acromial arch in this particular range of movement. A further test for this lesion is to ask the patient to take up the inclined walk standing position. Then, whilst retaining that trunk posture he is asked to elevate the arm. This is usually pain-free as the weight of the arm acts as a traction force on the shoulder joint and relieves the compression on the affected structures.

FROZEN SHOULDER
This is usually the result of a chronic state of this rotator cuff lesion, which has not been treated, thus allowing a chronic capsulitis of the shoulder joint to develop. Few patients willingly inflict pain on them-

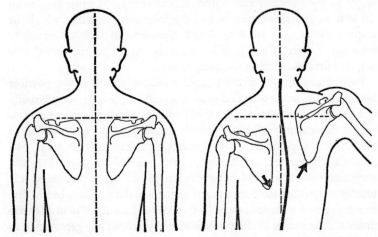

Fig. 7/1 To illustrate reverse scapulohumeral movement. Attempted abduction of the arm results in elevation of the scapula instead of rotation.

selves and therefore they avoid the painful arc of movement. They use the arm only for actions which involve a small range of pain-free movements of the shoulder and this range gradually becomes less as the capsule becomes thickened and adherent. In a few weeks there can be a complete loss of range, which is difficult, if not impossible to regain.

Consideration of all the findings and history should enable the examiner to make a differential diagnosis and so select the appropriate treatment. However, in the acute stage of shoulder lesions this may not be possible, and a diagnosis indicating an area of damage rather than a specific structure may well have to be made.

An established frozen shoulder may well be pain-free as all movements in the joint have ceased. Assessment of this condition should be made from the rear of the patient, from where it may be seen that the shoulder girdle rises as the arm abducts and no movement between the scapula and humerus can be detected because the structures move as one (see Fig. 7/2, below). A further test is to ask the patient to stand with his arms by his side, then to bend both elbows to a right angle. Keeping his upper arms close to his chest wall outward rotation is

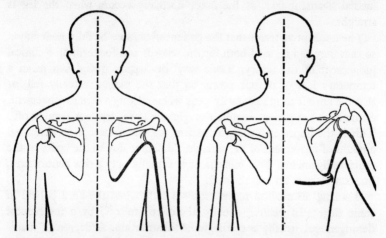

Fig. 7/2 Frozen shoulder. Attempted abduction of the arm results in 30° of lateral movement of the scapula. The distance between the humerus and the inferior angle of the scapula remains the same.

attempted. The frozen shoulder will only move a few degrees, and this is not true shoulder joint rotation. It is made by the action of trapezius and the rhomboid muscles retracting the scapula.

Mobility is the chief requirement of the shoulder region, but while full range movement is the aim of physiotherapy, this may well have to be compromised in order to obtain a pain-free, functional arm, especially if the patient is in the older age-group.

EXAMINATION OF THE KNEE

History

The time spent talking to a patient about how and when the incident occurred is most valuable. It will become obvious what tissues are likely to have been damaged, and to what extent, by the patient's remarks. A sensible patient can help greatly in the assessment of his injury. For example, a footballer may say that he was dribbling the ball in a forward direction, when he was tackled by another player. Immediately he attempted to pivot with his knee slightly flexed, but his foot was held in the tackle and so he sustained a rotational strain of his knee joint. This indicates that it is more likely to be a cartilage injury than a medial ligament tear, as the latter normally occurs when the leg is straight.

The descriptive terms that the patient uses must be fully understood so that they can be used both for the records and for forming a clinical judgement of the injury. 'Gave way' or 'letting down' can mean a temporary loss of muscle power so that the patient actually fell, or that the knee feels momentarily weak when making a certain movement. Sometimes the patient says he thought the lower leg 'was coming off'. This is the impression that the patient has when there is an abnormal amount of movement of the tibia on the femur due to the laxity of the cruciate ligaments. This movement is actually only a few centimetres, but can be seen on examination.

'Locking' in medical terms means a state when the knee is held in some degree of flexion, usually about 10° to 15°, by a mechanical derangement, usually a cartilaginous obstruction. A degree of manipulation, whether by the patient himself or another person, will be needed to unlock the knee joint. Many patients use the term 'locking' to describe a painful reluctance to move, combined with muscle spasm; or a momentary spasm of pain which checked movement.

'Lumps' or 'swellings' are terms used indiscriminately to describe either bony, soft tissue or fluid alterations that the patient feels when palpating his knee. Only by careful questioning can such remarks be helpful in diagnosis. A patient who has dislocated his patella seldom remarks on the patella being displaced, but complains of a lump which appears on the side of his knee. This is really the exposure of the medial condyle of the femur. Other patients are good historians and can clearly indicate where and how they feel a loose body, or a tag of cartilage which moves so that it can only be felt at certain times, or after certain movements.

Observation

It is useful to watch a patient unobtrusively as he enters a cubicle and gets onto an examination couch. The position of the knee joint when it bears weight, whether the patient 'swings' the leg up on the couch or has to assist it with his hands, the expression on his face at the time, all help to make a clinical assessment. The degree of flexion that the knee is held in while walking may gradually lessen as the patient relaxes on the couch. Any skin discoloration or alteration in contour should be noted.

Palpation

This allows the patient to get accustomed to his painful joint being handled, and if it is done with care, he will relax more easily since he does not feel so apprehensive. To the examiner it is an opportunity to feel the swelling and warmth of an inflammatory lesion and to feel the alteration in muscle tone when tenderness is present, thus helping to determine the site of the lesion.

Movement

Usually the patient is asked to demonstrate the degree of flexion and extension he is able to perform. A comparison of the muscle power of the unaffected and affected leg is made. Thereafter much of the examination is passive movement performed by the examiner to form the diagnosis. Many of these tests are performed on the sound leg first. This not only allows the patient to know what is going to be performed, but more importantly it gives a comparison of movement. All joints have some laxity and it is reasonable to assume that normally it is equal in a similar joint of the same patient, unless there is some obvious reason why this should not be so.

Ligament damage

TIBIAL COLLATERAL LIGAMENT

Medial ligament damage is tested with the knee extended (*not* hyperextended) and the joint is stabilized by the palm of the examiner's hand being placed on the lateral aspect of the knee with the fingers supporting the knee posteriorly. The other hand which is placed on the medial aspect of the lower tibia then abducts the tibia on the femur. If there is damage to the ligament the movement will be more than normal and pain will be felt by the patient, either on the medial condyle of the femur or along the upper tibia, depending on which end of the ligament has been damaged. The pain and muscle spasm are usually too great for this test to be conclusive diagnostically for a complete rupture of the ligament, and it may have to be repeated under an anaesthetic.

FIBULAR COLLATERAL LIGAMENT

Lateral ligament damage is tested by a similar method with the supporting hand held medially and the tibia adducted on the femur.

An alternative test can be performed with the patient in prone lying. The affected knee is flexed to 90°. The patient is then asked to relax and the operator holds the leg at the ankle and gives a slight lift which opens the knee joint (i.e. traction). The tibia is then rotated and if pain is experienced by the patient it is indicative of collateral ligament damage. (Only a few patients with severe damage will be able to flex their knee to a right angle in the acute stage.)

CRUCIATE LIGAMENT DAMAGE

When an anterior cruciate ligament is torn off violently it often removes a flake of bone and this is visible on an X-ray. The test for laxity is only possible if the patient can relax his knee completely. It is not conclusive evidence of a complete rupture. The hip and knee are flexed to 90°. The foot is rested on the couch and stabilized by the examiner lightly sitting on it. The examiner's hands are then placed around the tibial condyles so that the thumbs are either side of the tibial tubercle. The upper end of the tibia is then rocked forwards and back and the range is assessed against that of the other knee.

LIGAMENTUM PATELLAE DAMAGE

The leg is relaxed in the extended position and palpation will reveal the 'gap' either below or above the patella. (See Muscle Rupture, page 229.)

DAMAGE TO THE MENISCUS

When the knee is flexed to 90° palpation of the joint line will often elicit acute pain over a tear of the rim of the cartilage, or the tag may be felt. The test as for cruciate ligament laxity is performed, and may elicit pain which could indicate that a torn section of the meniscus is folded backward into the joint, causing strain on the anterior cruciate ligament. A 'springing' of the knee joint, that is gentle forced hyperextension of a knee that is held in slight flexion by spasm, can be helpful as an aid to diagnosis of a tear of the posterior horn of a cartilage, but it is performed with care as it may well be putting strain on the cruciate ligaments, which may be already under strain by the internal derangement of the joint.

McMurray's test

This is to confirm a meniscus lesion. The knee and hip are fully flexed. The examiner's hand is placed posteriorly round the knee joint so that the thumb and forefinger are on the joint line. The heel is gripped by the other hand and the tibia is rotated outward. A low-pitched clunk indicates a medial cartilage tear. The rotating of the tibia inwards would be performed to test a lateral cartilage. If no sound is obtained the procedure is repeated with the knee in less flexion. The less flexion needed to obtain the sound, the further inwards the tear. If no sound can be obtained then the manipulation is repeated when moving the knee through flexion or extension. It is often impossible to be certain where the tear is, or whether there is one, until an operation has been performed.

An alternative test is similar to that described for collateral ligaments. Again the patient is lying prone and flexes the knee to 90°. The operator holds the ankle and the patient is asked to relax. Pressure is then exerted to close the knee joint (compression) and the tibia is rotated. This grinding action causes pain if there is damage to the meniscus.

Patella tap

This test is used to establish if there is fluid in the knee joint. The knee is supported in a relaxed extended position. The operator then places his hand above the knee joint. This hand is then moved distally whilst exerting some posterior pressure, so that any fluid within the capsule is compressed. Whilst the position of this hand is maintained, the other is used to depress, or tap the patella against the femur. A knocking sound can be heard and felt when there is an effusion in the joint. Sometimes there is too much, or too little fluid to elicit the tap. An alternative procedure is to place both hands across the knee, one above and one below the patella. The fingers should be on one aspect and the thumbs on the other. Pressure is then exerted on the side of the joint by the fingers and if there is an effusion, the fluid will move away from the pressure and can be felt by the thumbs on the opposite side of the joint. The fluid's movement can also be observed.

EXAMINATION OF THE LOW BACK

History

Careful questioning of the patient is essential. It is important to understand what he means by the terms he uses to describe his pain and how it occurred, and to find out about previous incidents of trauma that he may not think of mentioning. For example most people over 40 have suffered some pain in the back before the incident which finally brings them to hospital. Questioning will elicit which time of day this was usually at its worst, and whether it stopped them from working, etc. A pain on waking is often an indication that there is a lack of mobility in the spine. Such pain 'wears off' as the patient moves about. Increasing pain and stiffness as the day progresses indicates a more inflammatory state which is caused by increasing protective muscle spasm.

A person who gives a history of a blow on his back will have local swelling, tenderness, etc., associated with a contusion at the site of the injury. The examination will be to determine the severity of injury and to exclude complications such as bony damage or damage to internal organs.

Observation

The way a patient walks or moves himself on arrival is always watched carefully since it is the only really free movement he will make. This observation is continued to include how he gets himself on or off a plinth, but this is not such valuable evidence as his first free movements. Thereafter he will be performing actions on request and these may not give a true picture.

POSTURE

This is always a most valuable guide to the severity of nerve root irritation. Unless there is a medical reason to make it impossible, the patient should always be examined standing. Any alteration of lumbar, thoracic or cervical curves should be observed from both the side and the rear of the patient. Any scoliosis and the relative position of the shoulders to the hips should be assessed from the back of the patient. The distribution of the muscle spasm should also be noted.

Palpation

Palpation of the back is an important part of the examination, because much can be deduced from the distribution of increased muscle tension. The patient stands with his back to the examiner, who places her flattened hands over the lower lumbar region. The difference in tension of the erector spinae muscles on each side can then be detected.

By gentle palpation, the whole lower back can be examined in order to ascertain the distribution of muscle spasm and its effect on the position of the vertebral column. The most usual pattern of muscle spasm is such that the vertebrae adjacent to the lesion are deviated to that side, with a compensatory muscle spasm above and on the opposite side, resulting in scoliosis.

Tenderness should be carefully noted. In many lesions, whilst the pain may be diffuse, there will be an area of localized tenderness which indicates the precise site of the lesion.

Movements

FORWARD FLEXION
The patient is asked to bend forward without bending his knees, and the muscle spasm evoked is carefully noted. If one knee were allowed to bend, the distribution of muscle spasm in the back would be altered and the effectiveness of the test nullified. During forward flexion, it is usual for the examiner to put her hand sideways over the spine so that the thumb and little finger touch the patient over the sacrum and upper lumbar vertebrae. Contact is maintained as the movement is performed and any alteration in distance between the digits is noted. If the distance shortens, which is rare, it would indicate extra spasm, and lengthening would indicate a degree of movement occurring in the lumbar spine. Such movement is not usual in an acute lesion. If the lesion is of lower lumbar origin, the hamstrings will go into spasm. The ability to 'touch the toes' has no bearing on the progress or severity of the condition.

Some patients will be able to touch their toes whilst their upper lumbar muscles are in severe spasm, others with no spasm will never be able to demonstrate this action. It is only a guide to the length of the hamstring muscles, and many chronic back sufferers will have gradually stretched the hamstrings to compensate for loss of lumbar flexion. Whilst this forward flexion is being attempted the patient is asked to indicate when and where pain is produced; this helps to determine the mechanism involved in the production of pain.

HYPEREXTENSION
Extension of the spine is then requested into the hyperextended position. In an acute lesion of the lower lumbar region this can seldom be performed as a posterolateral disc protrusion commonly occurs. However, if the disc had protruded anteriorly, hyperextension would be the post-traumatic stance and forward flexion would probably only be to the upright.

LATERAL FLEXION
This is not usually affected except that muscles involved in the action may be in spasm.

Lasègue's sign

When this was originally described by Lasègue he said that the patient should be lying relaxed in a supine position. The affected leg was then passively raised so that the hip and knee were each in flexion to 90°. Then keeping the hip still, the lower leg was raised to the straight position. If pain was experienced the test was described as positive. Today this test is usually adapted to a passive straight leg-raising which is performed slowly and carefully. During the first 30° of this movement no lumbar spine movement occurs, thereafter there is some movement, particularly at the level of L5 and stretching of the nerve root occurs. The nerve root movement is at its greatest when the leg is raised to between 60° and 80° (see Fig. 7/3, p. 219). The clinical interpretation of this sign is that if the pain is severe the lesion is likely to be the fifth lumbar nerve root.

Charnley is of the opinion that this test does not necessarily indicate a disc protrusion unless the back is stiff. He suggests a modification of the

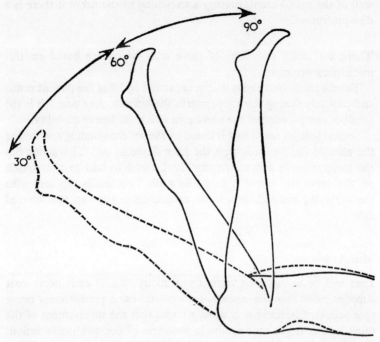

Fig. 7/3 To illustrate the significance of pain at certain points of straight leg-raising. 0°–30° usually pain-free. 30°–60° acute nerve irritation. 60°–90° sub-acute or mild nerve irritation.

test which is passive straight leg-raising until there is pain. Then flex the knee until the pain goes, and press sharply in the popliteal fossa without moving the hip or knee. If pain is elicited by this finger pressure it is a nerve root pain and not a muscular one.

Fajersztajn's sign

This is the name given after an Austrian neurologist found that when the non-affected leg is passively raised, pain is felt on the affected side. Woodhall and Hayes many years later were able to describe why this occurred. It is because when the leg is raised the lower lumbar nerve roots on the opposite side emerge a little from their foramina, shifting a little towards the middle line and to a lesser extent towards the anterior wall of the spinal canal, causing a stretching of the nerve if there is a disc protrusion.

There are many variations of these tests which are based on this mechanical principle.

Third lumbar nerve root lesions are tested by lying the patient prone and passively flexing the knee towards the buttock. Any pain felt is the result of compression of the nerve root due to its loss of mobility.

Second lumbar nerve root is tested by the patient standing and raising the affected leg forwards with the knee flexed to 90°. This action has the greatest nerve root movement for L2 and to add to the stretch on the nerve the trunk is flexed forward. This test is repeated with the other leg and will, to a lesser extent, cause pain on the affected side.

Muscle power

Loss will be assessed by static contractions. Whilst each nerve root supplies more than one muscle, each muscle has a predominant nerve root supply. Clinically it is usually found that the involvement of the third lumbar nerve root results in weakness of the quadriceps action, the fifth lumbar nerve root the extensors of the great toe, and the first sacral nerve root the gastrocnemius.

Sensory loss

Sensory loss will be assessed, but this, whilst following the pattern of the appropriate dermatome, is very variable from one patient to another. However, a reasonable guide is that L4 nerve root affects the area around the anteromedial aspect of the knee, L5 nerve root the dorsum of the foot, especially the great toe, and S1 nerve root the heel and lateral aspect of the foot.

Reflexes

These will also be tested. The loss of the patellar reflex would indicate an L3 nerve root and the loss of the plantar reflex an S1 nerve root involvement.

Nerve root	Reflexes		Muscles pre-dominantly affected	Areas of most usual sensation alteration
	Knee jerk	Ankle jerk		
L3	−	+	Quadriceps	
L4	+	+		Anteromedial aspect of knee
L5	+	+	Extensor of great toe	Dorsum of foot and great toe
S1	+	−	Gastrocnemius	Heel and lateral aspect of foot

SYNOVITIS

This term is used to describe an inflammation of the synovial membrane of a joint. When the synovium is injured excessive synovial fluid is secreted into the joint cavity. The quantity is dependent on the amount of trauma that has occurred, but it is not uncommon to find that the capsule is fully distended by this effusion. If the trauma has caused damage to blood vessels, the effusion will be bloodstained.

The most usual way to damage the synovium is a twisting strain on a joint, and this occurs most readily when the joint is flexed. It can be due to a direct blow. In either case other soft tissue damage may have occurred at the same time.

Let us take as an example traumatic synovitis of the knee which may have occurred as a result of an accident on a rugger field two hours previously.

CLINICAL FINDINGS

The knee joint is grossly swollen, clearly outlining the limits of the synovial membrane.

The leg is held in slight flexion (20°) so that the tension on the capsule and ligaments is reduced to a minimum. There is considerable muscle spasm of the hamstrings with inhibition of the quadriceps.

On palpation the joint is warm and the swelling is found to fluctuate. It is exquisitely tender.

Any movement of the joint causes great pain. It is for this reason that the player with a severe synovial injury cannot continue playing and is often carried off the field.

INVESTIGATION

It is essential that a very thorough investigation is made. An X-ray should be considered to eliminate the possibility of damage to the joint surfaces. Assessment for ligamentous damage may be prevented by the extreme pain, and examination under anaesthetic with X-ray control will have to be considered.

TREATMENT

Only very occasionally is the joint tension so severe that the effusion needs to be aspirated. The danger of infection is so high that this is seldom performed and then only with full aseptic precautions.

When all other major damage has been excluded the knee is usually supported by a pressure bandage. Whilst this may be able to prevent further effusion it will not aid the resolution of the existing one. It should not be retained for more than three days.

Ice therapy is most helpful, as is deep heat for assisting in the quick absorption of the effusion.

Muscle activity, within the limits of pain-free movement, should be started at once.

Whilst the joint is warm and tense, that is, showing the signs of acute inflammation, excess movement would result in exacerbation of the lesion. However, the muscle contractions will help to control the effusion and prevent muscle atrophy which occurs very quickly in the quadriceps due to the inhibiting factor of the spasm of the hamstring group. The rule should be for the patient to be taught a few simple exercises to do at home for five minutes in every hour. It must be remembered that the athlete or sportsman will always overdo exercises and suitable warnings should be given. The most important exercise, and one which cannot be performed too often, is full extension of the knee joint to the locked position. This involves the vastus medialis muscle in the last part of the movement. This muscle atrophies quickly and is more difficult to re-educate at a later stage of treatment, so that it is important to restore its function immediately.

At first all exercises should be performed in the non-weight-bearing posture. No walking should be allowed on a knee that exhibits a quadriceps lag on straight leg-raising; but of course the patient will be allowed to walk with crutches, taking no weight on the affected leg.

It must be remembered that the sportsman will soon become generally out of training when he is restricted to non-weight-bearing exercises and a general 'whole body' programme of exercises should be given as well as specific knee exercises. There is, for instance, no reason why he should not go swimming or use a static rowing machine with the affected leg left to the side.

Weight-bearing exercises will probably begin at about two weeks if the injury has been severe. These will be progressed to form the basis of an early full training programme. It is essential that absolutely full fitness and confidence is restored before play is allowed.

PROGNOSIS
Normally the function and power of the knee should have been fully restored, so that the player can participate in his sport again, within three to four weeks.

TENOSYNOVITIS

This is an inflammation of the tendon sheath which can be caused by a sudden wrench or a direct blow, though it usually occurs as a result of over-use. The effusion thus caused reduces the lumen of the sheath so making it more difficult for the tendon to run freely. This is an acute tenosynovitis which can, if repeated, become a chronic state in which the continuous process of fibrotic repair makes a thickened sheath, with tiny fibroid nodules, often referred to as melon-seed bodies. This loss of normal lumen makes all movements of the tendon painful.

Any tendon sheath can be affected, but some are more vulnerable to the effects of over-use than others, because of the mechanics of their anatomical action. An example of this is the common sheath for extensor pollicis brevis and abductor pollicis longus which have an angular pull as they pass around the radial styloid. Acute tenosynovitis of this sheath is known as de Quervain's disease.

De Quervain's disease (example)

Women are affected more often than men. The patient will probably give a history of having just started a new job in a factory. The work involves a light gripping action, which has to be repeated constantly several times a minute. After two days at this work she woke to find she could not move her thumb because of the pain.

CLINICAL PICTURE

There is a localized sausage-shaped swelling over the inflamed tendon sheath, which is very warm and tender.

Any movement of the tendon within the sheath causes pain. The pain may be so great that movement appears impossible. It has often been found that these patients have a low pain tolerance and will be disinclined to move any part of the hand or even the forearm.

IMMEDIATE TREATMENT

The thumb and wrist are rested on a cock-up splint. This is to restrict movement rather than prevent it.

To obtain a quick absorption of the inflammation, ultrasound and ice therapy, or shortwave diathermy may be used. No movement of the tendons involved is encouraged for the first two days.

PROGRESSION

Once the very acute pain has subsided, unresisted movements are added. At first these will only be performed for a minute several times a day, using the splint for rest at other times.

After about seven to ten days, free gentle use of the hand will be encouraged with gradually shortening periods of rest on the splint. It is often useful to retain the splint for use at night for rather longer than it will be required for use during the day.

Before the patient is allowed to return to her job, a simulated gripping device must be found for her to practise upon. This serves several purposes:

It can determine whether the inflammatory state has resolved.

It can be used to check that the patient is performing the action of gripping properly. It is often found that these patients are only using the thumb to make the grip against statically held fingers. By encouraging them to share the work-load by actively flexing the fingers, further incidents may be prevented. A repetition of similar trauma may lead to a chronic inflammation of the tendon sheath.

It will prove to the patient that she can have confidence in her ability to use her hand effectively at work.

Sportsmen seldom get de Quervain's disease but they do get tenosynovitis affecting the biceps, or the flexors of the fingers. This latter can either affect the common sheath in the region of the carpal bones, or more likely, in the digital synovial sheath.

Chronic tenosynovitis

This is usually treated with an infiltration of hydrocortisone and a resting plaster, which is retained until there is complete resolution (ten to twelve days). Occasionally transverse frictions are requested after the plaster has been removed. Persistent lesions may require an operation to relieve the symptoms. It is seldom that these patients require physiotherapy as they use their limb normally once the pain has subsided.

BURSITIS

Bursae are small membranous sacs lined by synovium, which are sited to prevent frictional wear on tendons at joints. This friction could be between two tendons, but more usually it is between a tendon and a bone. True bursae are found at certain joints such as the elbow, heel and knee, but it is also possible to form a bursa over a joint which has become damaged or deformed and presents a new area of friction for a tendon. These are called adventitious bursae, but their reaction to injury is the same as that of a true bursa.

An acute bursitis is caused by a direct blow such as a fall on the knee or shoulder, or it can be the result of too much activity, especially of an unaccustomed action. Many bursae can be injured and cause little discomfort to the patient, since pain only occurs if pressure is put on to the inflamed bursa. For example, olecranon bursitis is almost painless until the elbow is leant upon. However, the subacromial bursa, when inflamed, is acutely painful due to the pressures put upon it during movements of the shoulder joint.

Subacromial bursitis (example)

A middle-aged patient wakes up to find he has a very painful shoulder. The day before he had been decorating a ceiling, a job he is not accustomed to doing.

CLINICAL PICTURE
He will be holding his arm close to his body, usually supporting the elbow with his other hand.

Any movement will cause great pain and he will have difficulty in removing his clothes.

It will be found that he has spasm of the adductor and medial rotator muscles of his shoulder, with a very tender area along the lateral border of the acromion.

The area will feel warm, but little swelling will be present as the damaged tissues are confined within the bursa and this is deep to the middle fibres of deltoid.

IMMEDIATE TREATMENT
After suitable investigation to eliminate other pathology, his arm will be rested in a sling under his clothes. Physiotherapy will aim at relieving the pain and reducing the inflammation.

PROGRESSION
It is important to retain shoulder movements. After the very acute phase is over, assisted movements must be given. These are progressed to full active movements as the inflammation resolves.

The anatomical construction of a shoulder is so complex that it is often impossible to decide which structures are damaged. However, the treatment is the same for all soft tissue lesions of the shoulder rotator cuff.

Whilst a sling may be worn for a few days, it must not be retained for longer, especially in the older age-group, or range will be lost which it may not be possible to regain. For this reason full range movements must be aimed for at a very early stage. Ice therapy will usually relieve the pain and muscle spasm to enable P.N.F. (proprioceptive neuromuscular facilitation) techniques to be used to build up the power and range of movement. Functional activity is given as soon as possible.

For Bibliography see end of Chapter 11, p. 291.

CHAPTER 8

Injuries to Soft Tissues II

by M. K. PATRICK, OBE, MCSP, SRP

INJURIES TO MUSCLES AND TENDONS

These injuries range from a simple strain to a complete rupture of the muscle or tendon. Within this range come some of the most common injuries sustained by athletes and sportsmen as well as the general public.

Strain of muscle

Normal muscle is able to respond to the demands made upon it and is capable of a graded contraction directly proportional to the stress. It is only capable of this response if all the components of the neuromuscular mechanism are working co-ordinately. If a sudden stretching force is applied to a muscle unexpectedly, the response may not be sufficiently co-ordinated and the result may be a rupture of a few muscle fibres or a minor tear in the connective tissue framework of the muscle.

Such injuries happen to athletes and sportsmen at the beginning of the season before they are fully trained, or to members of the general public who try to perform an action beyond their muscle strength. The effect of the damage will be seen at the weakest point in the muscle, and usually in muscles which work over two joints. The terms 'strain', 'tear' or 'pull' of muscle are commonly used to indicate a relatively trivial injury. The amount of haemorrhage that occurs will be directly proportional to the vascularity of the muscle and inversely proportional to its tone. The haematoma lies in the extracellular and interstitial spaces.

227

CLINICAL FEATURES

The patient presents with a muscle which has a localized tender swelling at the point of injury.

Protective muscle spasm and pain will be demonstrated proportional to the severity of the injury.

These will cause limitation of movement.

TREATMENT

Ice therapy (that is a pad soaked in ice-cold water, not direct ice), is the first-aid treatment for this injury. Usually strapping is applied to the area more for reassurance than support, since the bleeding will be controlled by the compression that occurs as the intramuscular tension builds up. Physiotherapy is not required for the acute lesion, but may be needed to encourage the patient to regain confidence in the limb. Normally clotting takes place in a few hours and in about three days full activity can be undertaken without fear of further tissue damage.

Contusions

These are the results of a crush injury, or a direct blow or kick. The blood and lymph vessels in the connective tissues of the muscle framework are ruptured and their contents released into the surrounding tissues to form a haematoma. The result is similar to that described for muscle strain except that with extrinsic violence there is subcutaneous as well as deep connective tissue damage. The sheath of the muscle may well be ruptured, allowing a muscle hernia to develop. The example will be taken of a footballer who has received a kick on his thigh over rectus femoris about 9 inches (23 cm) above the knee joint and slightly lateral to mid-line, two hours previous to examination.

CLINICAL FEATURES

The leg will be held in slight flexion due to the protective spasm of the hamstrings. The quadriceps will show inhibition and loss of tone except in the vicinity of the injury where muscle fibres will be in spasm.

A marked swelling over the site of injury.

This swelling will be both warm and tender.

TREATMENT

Ice-cold pads applied over the site of injury are the first-aid treatment for these lesions and may be continued for several days if required.

Strapping is applied, usually either over a cotton cylindrical bandage, or reversed, so that it does not adhere to the skin. The leg should be elevated to assist drainage whilst physiotherapy is given and the patient instructed to elevate his leg at home. Ultrasound therapy given to the area proximal to the haematoma aids rapid resolution. Static quadriceps exercises are most important in that they restore the tone to the muscle and aid the reabsorption of the haematoma.

PROGRESSION

Due to the dangers of further damage to the blood vessels knee movements are usually delayed for 24 to 48 hours in severe injuries. Thereafter gentle knee movements are encouraged, watching always for any increase in bleeding. This would be indicated by an increase in both pain and swelling. These exercises are performed with a supporting bandage on.

The maximum effect of ultrasound and ice therapy is obtained during the first week. If further treatment is necessary then shortwave diathermy may be given. At this stage there should be discoloration of the skin distal to the injured area. If there is not it may indicate that the haematoma has become 'trapped' by the organization of the exudate peripherally, thus preventing its drainage. This can soon lead to ulceration and medical advice should be sought, as aspiration may be necessary.

Usually progress is quite fast after the first ten days and is similar to that of muscle strain. The type of exercise is more fully described under Synovitis of the Knee (p. 221).

The long-term complication of severe haematoma is calcification within the muscle. If this causes weakness or loss of movement, the calcified mass may be removed surgically some months later.

Rupture of a muscle

A complete rupture of a muscle belly rarely occurs except as a result of laceration, and the surgeon will have to consider the need or desirability of suture. Spontaneous repair will not take place as the two parts of the muscle contract, leaving a wide gap. Partial ruptures are more common and have been described under Contusions (p. 228). A complete rupture can occur as a result of a direct blow on a contracted muscle, or by forced stretching of an already contracted one.

Such a complete tear of the belly of a muscle can occur in a very fit young athlete, and the belly of the rectus femoris is most often affected. A similar strain in an elderly person would result in a tear of the quadriceps femoris tendon immediately above the upper pole of the patella. In those who are neither elderly nor highly trained athletes, the rectus pull would tear the tendon below the patella.

Let us take as an example a young athlete who has sustained a complete rupture of rectus femoris an hour previously.

CLINICAL FEATURES

A flexed knee due to the spasm of the hamstrings which are only weakly opposed.

A large swollen area over the site of the injury which is very warm and fluctuates on palpation. This is a haematoma and is tender.

The upper section of rectus is contracted upwards and the lower section downwards to form hard 'knots' of muscle, leaving a palpable gap between them.

IMMEDIATE TREATMENT

The two ends of the muscle are brought together and repaired surgically.

The leg is supported in a back-splint for 10 to 21 days. During this time static quadriceps exercises are given and active knee flexion is usually encouraged after the tenth day.

PROGRESSION

This is as for partial tear or severe contusion, once the surgeon has agreed to the starting of knee flexion and weight-bearing.

Rupture of tendons

The causes of these injuries are the same as for ruptures of the muscle tissue.

A completely torn tendon will not repair itself spontaneously. Whether the surgeon decides to effect a surgical repair will largely depend on the age of the patient and the disability caused by the injury. For example, it is not uncommon for the tendon of the long head of the biceps to rupture in the over-70 age-group. This is seldom operated upon since the disability is a weakening of flexion of the elbow, but not a loss of the action, and does not usually warrant surgical intervention. However, complete rupture of a tendo-calcaneus causes great disability and the tendon is usually sutured.

EXAMPLE ONE
An elderly man with a ruptured long head of biceps tendon.

The patient will probably explain that he suddenly found difficulty in using his arm when he was trying to put his arm inside the sleeve of his coat. A history of traumatic incident can seldom be given.

CLINICAL APPEARANCE
The belly of the muscle will have contracted down into a hard knot, leaving a clearly defined 'space' where it would normally lie. This is even more clearly demonstrated if the elbow is flexed against slight resistance.

If it is truly the tendon that has ruptured, as is usual in the elderly, there is little swelling or bruising since the exudation is minimal. If, however, the tendon ruptures at the union with the muscle, the blood content of the exudate is increased.

IMMEDIATE TREATMENT
Rest in a large arm sling will be given, but active movements of the shoulder and elbow must be encouraged at once or range will be lost, and this may never be fully regained. A full range of movement of shoulder, elbow and radio-ulnar joints must be given, even if they have to be assisted or passively performed once on the first day. Relaxation of muscle spasm is needed to obtain pain relief and this is best obtained by resisted movements of the antagonist group. Heat is usually helpful. If there is a large haematoma or effusion then the techniques previously described under Contusions (p. 228) may be tried.

The sling must be removed totally by the second or third day or flexion contracture of the elbow will develop as the torn muscle becomes adherent. To prevent spasm the hand can be carried some of the time in a coat pocket or the elbow rested on a chair-arm or table. Active use of the arm should be practised in the physiotherapy department to show the patient that it can be used normally. It is advisable to keep these patients in the department for most of the day in the first week after injury so that they can have repeated short activity sessions. If left at home they tend not to use the arm.

Full but weakened function should be obtained in two to three weeks.

EXAMPLE TWO

A ruptured tendo-calcaneus.

A fit, middle-aged man has torn his tendo-calcaneus when doing a sudden inco-ordinate muscle movement involving a powerful plantar-flexion of the foot. Most commonly this is done in sport, but it can be done by stepping onto the edge of a kerb instead of fully onto the pavement. The foot, instead of being stopped at 90°, is forced into full dorsiflexion. The calf muscle makes a violent contraction to try to counteract the dorsiflexion, but is unable to take the strain.

CLINICAL APPEARANCE

The belly of the gastrocnemius will be contracted upwards, but cannot retract far because the aponeurosis of the posterior aspect of the tendon is united to the soleus muscle, gradually forming a single tendon. However, a clearly defined gap in the tendon is palpable about one or two inches (2·5 to 5 cm) above the insertion into the calcaneum. Occasionally this is masked by a chronic thickening of the area or a local swelling.

Plantarflexion of the foot is performed weakly and only in a non-weight-bearing posture, by the posterior tibial muscles.

TREATMENT

The tendon is surgically repaired. The lower leg is put in plaster with the foot plantarflexed.

PROGRESSION

After about three to four weeks the foot is brought up to a right angle, and walking with crutches is permitted. At four to six weeks a removable cast is often used so that active non-weight-bearing exercises can be given and non-weight-bearing walking with crutches has to be resumed. At about six to eight weeks full weight-bearing walking is allowed. The patient should be warned at this stage not to allow his foot to be suddenly forced into dorsiflexion.

Graduated exercises are given to build up the power of the calf muscles which will have atrophied considerably. The final result depends on the patient's willingness to practise exercises, and his confidence in his own ability. Some patients make a very good recovery and are able to raise the body weight onto the ball of the affected foot. Others are not able to do this. A poor result is in part a reflection on the therapist who should have been able to build up the patient's enthusiasm and confidence throughout the rehabilitation period.

Partial ruptures of tendons are said by some surgeons to be impossible, that is the tendon either tears completely or does not tear at all. Other surgeons say partial ruptures can occur but do not require treatment beyond reassurance and perhaps an injection of local anaesthetic.

Peritendonitis

One of the most common injuries in athletics is peritendonitis of the tendo-calcaneus. When this is seen it is often an acute exacerbation of a chronic state and may exhibit stenosing or crepitus. The former will require operation, but the latter should resolve with rest. It is important that the rest period is at least ten days, during which time no heel raising should be performed. A pad in the heel of the shoe to elevate the heel, and walking with a shortened stride, will help to reduce the strain on the tendon. Any pain, however slight, should be taken to indicate that the activity must be reduced.

The physiotherapy needed is ultrasound and ice therapy, or short-wave diathermy during the rest period, to help speed the resolution of the inflammation. Thereafter a carefully controlled introduction to movement of the tendon should be made. Running and jumping exercises should not be attempted during the first three weeks. Full training should be delayed until there is no pain on plantarflexion in weight-bearing or jumping. This is probably five or six weeks after the incident. Any attempt to hurry back to athletics before the condition is completely resolved will result in a recurrence which is not only painful, but undermines the confidence of the athlete in his future ability.

LIGAMENTOUS DAMAGE

Normally a joint is stabilized by the muscles which control its movements, but if a strong external force is applied to the joint, particularly if it occurs unexpectedly as in an accident, the ligaments will be stretched. The individual fibres of the ligament will either tolerate the stress or rupture. The proportion of the fibres ruptured determines the clinical findings, the treatment required and the terminology used to describe the injury.

In the following text, the classification used by Williams in *Sports Medicine* is followed:

'Stretched ligament': an occasional fibre ruptured.

'Mild sprain': a small proportion of fibres ruptured.

'Severe sprain': about half the fibres are ruptured.

'Complete rupture of the ligament': all fibres ruptured.

It must be remembered that other soft tissue damage must have taken place in all but the mildest of injuries, and probably in these too. The doctor and physiotherapist must assess the total clinical evidence and base treatment on their findings.

EXAMPLE ONE
Stretched ligament.

This might be presented by a patient who complains of having stumbled, and in preventing his fall has taken the force of the body weight on the medial border of the hand. The ulnar collateral ligament is stretched.

CLINICAL FINDINGS
A small swelling over the ulnocarpal joint, the pain of which limits movement, particularly radial deviation.

TREATMENT
Usually Elastoplast strapping for a week and full activity is all that is required.

EXAMPLE TWO
Mild sprain.

This might be presented by a housewife who says that whilst she was making a bed her thumb was caught in a sheet as she tucked the bedclothes in, and it was forcibly hyperextended. She may well have ruptured a few fibres of the palmar ligament of the metacarpophalangeal joint.

CLINICAL FINDINGS
The thumb is held in slight flexion.

The metacarpophalangeal joint is very slightly swollen on the palmar aspect and very tender over the area of the damaged ligamentous tissue.

Whilst all movements are possible, hyperextension of the thumb (i.e. a repeat of the direction of injury) causes acute pain.

IMMEDIATE TREATMENT
Ultrasound therapy or shortwave diathermy is given to the affected
area to help resolve the inflammation. Strapping in the form of a spica
is applied to give support. The patient is encouraged to use the hand
fully.

PROGRESSION
This should be fast, the strapping is removed at seven to ten days and
full power and function recovered within two weeks.

EXAMPLE THREE
Severe sprain.
A youth has sustained an inversion injury to the ankle on a rugger
field.

CLINICAL FINDINGS
The foot will be in slight plantarflexion with some protective spasm in
the peronei.
There will be an egg-shaped localized swelling over the anterior
talofibular ligament. This ligament is the most vulnerable because of
the natural rotation of the forefoot.
The site of the lesion will be warm and tender.
Within a few hours of the injury the swelling will become less clearly
defined and may well spread across the dorsum of the foot, and postero-
laterally around the ankle.
Inversion will be severely limited by pain and muscle spasm.
Other movements will be performed in small range only.
X-ray investigation should be given to exclude bony injury.

TREATMENT
Since the ligament is not completely torn, conservative treatment will
be required. The speed of starting physiotherapy is very important.
Ultrasound and ice therapy should be given at once with the limb elevated. These are followed immediately by the application of a stirrup-
type Elastoplast strapping which holds the foot in eversion. Since the
strapping has to be removed frequently, it is usual to shave the limb
first. Walking, with two sticks if need be, should be started at once, but
the patient should only take short strides in order to eliminate a limp.
After the first few steps the pain eases off. It is very important that

walking is practised for short periods throughout the day. Progress in activity should be made quite quickly, but care must be taken to ensure that weight-bearing on an inverted foot does not take place for several weeks. For this reason the boy should be advised not to play rugger for two months if the injury has been severe.

EXAMPLE FOUR

Complete rupture of a ligament.

This might be presented by a pedestrian, who was struck on the lateral aspect of his leg by a car bumper. At the moment of impact the leg was fully extended. The force was such that it momentarily forced open the medial aspect of the knee joint and the tibial collateral ligament ruptured.

CLINICAL FINDINGS

The leg will be held in slight flexion due to the protective spasm of the hamstring muscles.

Within an hour of the incident there will be an effusion of the whole knee joint.

Localized tenderness over the site of the lesion will be very marked in the early stages. This becomes masked with the passing of time and the increase of the general effusion.

All movements will be grossly restricted by pain and muscle spasm, making it difficult to determine the site of the actual lesion.

X-ray investigation will be required. This may show the elevation of a flake of bone from the tibia or femur if the rupture has occurred at either of these points. It is often necessary to examine the knee whilst the patient is under an anaesthetic. The knee joint is given manual stress to open the joint to determine if a complete rupture has occurred.

TREATMENT

Surgery is required to repair the ligament. The leg will then be enclosed in a plaster cylinder from groin to ankle. This is retained for four to six weeks. The patient is usually kept non-weight-bearing for the first 10 to 21 days depending on how easily the surgical repair was made. After this walking is permitted. Once the plaster is removed knee movements are begun. The knee is usually supported by a back-splint (i.e. posterior half of the plaster cylinder) until the therapist is sure that the muscle power is sufficiently restored to protect the ligament from stress.

Full range of movement and power should be restored in two to three months from the time of the injury.

Sprung back

Young fit sportsmen do not suffer disc lesions as a result of their activities unless there is a major catastrophe such as the collapse of a rugger scrum, or a novice weight-lifter attempting too heavy a lift. They do, however, sustain repeated minor trauma, which can lead to early disc degeneration. This is particularly true of high and long jumpers, hammer and disc-throwers. They are frequently subjected to flexion stresses manifested as muscle spasm which usually resolve spontaneously after a few days, particularly if they can 'relax' the tense muscles. For this reason heat and massage are sometimes given.

The term sprung back is often used in sport. It is really a sprain of the lumbar intervertebral ligaments. This can be so severe that there is instability (which is demonstrable on stress X-rays), allowing a disc protrusion. The repeated attacks of low back pain or sciatica that follow can mean the end of sport participation. Sprung back in its milder form is treated as any other ligament strain.

DAMAGE OF MENISCI AND MENISCECTOMY

The menisci of the knee joint serve several purposes. They act as 'shock absorbers' in the straight leg posture as when walking, and as 'rockers' for the rolling action of the femoral condyles during flexion or extension. They are usually injured by a rotation strain on a flexed knee whilst it is weight-bearing.

It is very unusual for a child to tear a cartilage, but it is possible. The young and middle-aged form the majority of patients who suffer from this injury in its traumatic form, that is to say the patient can give a definite history of sudden pain, loss of power and range, with 'locking' of the joint (see also p. 212 for Examination of the Knee Joint). In the over-60 age-group a meniscus can be torn without the patient being able to give a history of any definite injury. This is because the cartilage is somewhat degenerative and possibly has had many previous minor injuries. Finally a minor incident completes a tear, or moves an already torn tag (which may well have been folded back within the joint), into a position where it cannot be tolerated. In this age-group the cartilage, either in its entirety, or just the torn slip, will have to be removed, since spontaneous repair is unlikely.

In younger people it is not thought advisable to remove menisci unless they have given rise to several previous episodes and have become an intolerable handicap, or if the 'locking' does not respond to manipulation. If the meniscus is removed the knee joint is mechanically imperfect, for the replacement cartilage that grows does not have the correct contours for the rolling action of the condyles of the femur, and so the knee is slightly less stable because hyperextension can take place. This defect is largely overcome by good muscle power when the patient is young, but later in life it often gives rise to further problems.

CLINICAL PICTURE
Immediately the incident takes place the knee which was bent at the time of injury, will 'lock'. This is a combination of muscle spasm caused by pain as well as the actual mechanical obstruction of cartilage. Sometimes the knee will only stay in this position for a few minutes. Gradually the muscle spasm lessens and the knee recovers its normal degree of laxity so that it can slowly be eased to a straighter position. In some cases the knee cannot be straightened until it has been manipulated under an anaesthetic.

The knee will lack full extension and any attempt to 'spring' it to the extended or hyperextended position will cause pain and increase the muscle spasm in the hamstrings.

An acute synovitis of the knee joint will develop slowly over a period of a few hours. (See also Synovitis, p. 221.)

TREATMENT
Once the knee has been unlocked it is then rested for at least 24 hours in a compression bandage or on a back-splint. Static quadriceps exercises are started quickly to restore the lost tone of the muscles and to help to control the effusion by their compression action. As soon as the acute inflammation has subsided, muscle and joint activity is gradually increased. Full power and function must be obtained before the patient is discharged.

If full range and power cannot be obtained it may indicate that a 'tag' of torn cartilage is rolled back in the intercondylar notch, causing a strain on the anterior cruciate ligament when the knee is fully extended. This prevents the quadriceps muscles from performing their full action and the vastus medialis muscle will atrophy very quickly. If full flexion is not possible, this may indicate a posterior horn tear. These patients may well be ordered 'provocative exercises', that is exercises devised to reproduce similar strains to those which occurred at the time of the incident. These exercises are chosen to subject the knee joint to rotational stress with the knee in flexion and under load. Before these are given, it is important to explain to the patient the purpose of the exercises, otherwise if the knee does 'lock' and operation is decided upon, he may feel that the therapist was to blame. This could lead to a lack of confidence in the therapist's ability which would be detrimental at a later stage of rehabilitation.

AFTER MENISCECTOMY

The routine of postoperative treatment will depend on the surgeon. Usually the knee is supported in a compression bandage for at least a few days. Knee movements may be started on the second day, or not until the tenth day. The patient may be allowed to resume partial or complete weight-bearing at any time from a few days to ten days postoperatively. However, before the patient is allowed to bear weight it is important that he has good control of his quadriceps muscles and can perform a straight leg-raising without a quadriceps lag. Progress is usually uneventful, with full power and range at six weeks. It is important to remind the patient that the power of the quadriceps must be maintained or further incidents may occur.

The degree and type of rehabilitation required will depend on the age, activity and occupation of the patient. Miners, and others who work in flexed positions, are particularly at risk and require a very strong knee before a return to work can be allowed. In sport a meniscus lesion is a hazard of footballers and others, and careful, graded training must be undertaken before the resumption of competitive sport. Circuit training is a useful method of developing strength and endurance. (See Chapter 9, p. 253.)

DISLOCATIONS

Any joint may suffer a dislocation, that is one bone may be displaced out of its normal joint position. By their anatomical construction some joints are less stable than others and therefore dislocate more readily. This is especially true of the shoulder joint which has poorly adapted articular surfaces and no true ligaments to support the capsule. The hip joint, on the other hand, which is a similar type of joint, has deep acetabulum and strong ligaments and is not easily dislocated, except that a flexed hip dislocates relatively easily because the capsule is thin posteriorly and the head of the femur is not well supported in this position. This is an increasingly common injury in car accidents when the knee strikes the dashboard.

CATEGORIES OF DISLOCATION

(*i*) A complete dislocation when the dislocated bone is lying completely out of its normal position.

(*ii*) A subluxed, or partial, dislocation where the bone is out of its normal position but still in partial contact with the opposing joint surface.

(*iii*) A spontaneously reduced dislocation. This occurs when the bone has been dislocated momentarily and has sprung back into its normal position again.

When a joint is dislocated there must be soft tissue damage. The amount of this damage depends on two factors, the distance the bones have been separated and the structure of the joint involved.

For example, a shoulder joint which is not held rigidly by ligaments can, if the force is not too severe, be dislocated with a minimal stretching of the soft tissues, causing only slight damage. However, in a violent dislocation of the shoulder, when the humeral head is widely separated from the glenoid cavity, very severe soft tissue damage will be sustained. The capsule will be torn, ligaments stretched, even an avulsion fracture of the greater tuberosity may occur. Blood vessels, nerves and cartilaginous structures may also be damaged.

CLINICAL PICTURE

The physiotherapist is not required to diagnose or reduce dislocations.

However, the abnormal anatomical appearance of the joint affected would make the diagnosis obvious to her. This is especially true of shoulder dislocations. A close appraisal of the shoulders will reveal a gap, perhaps marked by an effusion, where the head of the humerus ought to be. It is often easier to feel this rather than to observe it. Subluxations are not always easily identified without an X-ray. In the elderly, who have a weak musculature, the inability to move the shoulder is often incorrectly attributed to soft tissue damage, when in fact they have a subluxed joint. Redislocation or subluxation can easily occur in these elderly patients and it is important for the physiotherapist to check for any malalignment each time the patient attends for treatment, especially in the first 10 days.

Effusion into and around the joint will always be present immediately after reduction.

There will also be some warmth, indicating the inflamed state of the joint. These two signs will vary according to the amount of soft tissue damage and are a very rough guide to the time that recovery is likely to take.

TREATMENT
The immediate treatment for completely dislocated or subluxed joints is reduction to replace the bone into its normal position. The quicker this can be done the less the signs of damage will be, as the soft tissues are no longer stretched. A finger joint that is dislocated and reduced within minutes of the injury will only be slightly swollen and tender for a day or two, but if it is left dislocated and the patient makes his way to hospital for a reduction, perhaps with a time lag of over an hour, then the finger will be very swollen and painful for perhaps as long as 10 days after the injury.

Obviously some joints cannot be reduced quickly. The reduction of the hip joint, for example, requires an anaesthetic to overcome the muscle spasm which follows the injury. It may be necessary to wait for several hours before it is safe to give the anaesthetic. The soft tissues around the joint which are being stretched while the joint is disorganized respond to this by pouring out exudate so that there is a large effusion and great pain on any movement, however slight.

The shoulder dislocation often happens on the sports field. 'Instant reduction' used to be carried out by another player. This practice has now been discontinued since a hastily performed reduction could well be a bad reduction, which caused more damage than the original injury. The availability of a 24-hour Accident and Emergency Service has made medical care readily available. Many of these patients have little pain or swelling after reduction.

The elderly person, who may fall at home onto the outstretched hand and dislocate his shoulder, may not realize what injury he has sustained. He is aware only that his shoulder is painful if he moves it. These people often wait to go to the doctor's surgery later in the day and from there to hospital. The delay before reduction may be many hours. By this time there will be a gross effusion and full recovery of function is often delayed by weeks.

Movement of the affected joint immediately after reduction is not advisable. However, it is important to ascertain that the joints adjacent to the injury move normally. Any lack of movement should be considered carefully to see if it might indicate a nerve injury. (Alteration of skin sensation would also indicate this.)

Immediately after reduction (i.e. on the day of the injury) there should not be any alteration in the skin colour distal to the injury. If there is any, a check should be made of the pulses to ascertain if the blood vessels are damaged. If there is any doubt medical advice must be sought at once.

Movement should be encouraged the following day. Any gross effusion, or complications such as nerve involvement, will be treated as for any other similar lesion. Except for the elderly, or patients with severe injury, physiotherapy is seldom needed for more than a few days. Ice therapy and P.N.F. (proprioceptive neuromuscular facilitation) are the most effective aids for regaining normal movements. The only complication that might occur is the formation of adhesions due to lack of full range movements.

INTERVERTEBRAL DISC LESIONS

The term 'disc lesion' is used to describe the effects of degeneration, rupture, 'slipping' or bulging of the disc as well as nerve root pain. Intervertebral discs are firmly attached to the surfaces of the bodies of the vertebrae above and below them, as well as to the anterior and posterior longitudinal ligaments. They are shaped to fit the opposing vertebrae and consist of an outer annulus and an inner nucleus. The annulus is made up of concentric lamellae, the outer layers of which are primarily fibrous and the inner ones fibrocartilaginous. The fibres of the annulus interlace with each other and resist the forces of rotation. The nucleus pulposus is placed nearer to the back than the front of the disc. It changes in structure from a soft mucoid gelatinous substance in the first decade of life to a soft fibrocartilage in later years; this is difficult to distinguish from the annulus.

The depth of the disc in comparison to the depth of the adjacent vertebrae determines the amount of movement possible between the segments. This vertebral body/disc ratio is greatest in the cervical region and least in the thoracic.

In the young adult the discs are so strong that it is more likely, when violence is applied to the spine, for the vertebra to be affected than for a healthy disc to be damaged.

The ageing process, coupled with wear and tear occasioned by movement (maximal in the cervical and lumbar regions), causes the rupture of some of the fibres of the annulus, and when this has occurred the disc can become internally or externally displaced. Since the annulus is weaker in construction posterolaterally, this is the usual area to show the first signs of degeneration.

The shape of the disc contributes to the curvature of the spine. The lumbar and cervical curves develop as secondary curves and are therefore convex forwards. To allow for this the discs in these regions are wedge-shaped, thicker in front than behind. Flexion compresses the anterior surface of the disc. This will tend to cause further backward displacement of nuclear material through the cracked fibres of the annulus where the structure has been previously weakened. This can lead to a posterior protrusion of the disc into the vertebral canal.

In the lumbar region there is extra compression on the discs because of the greater body weight transmitted through them and because the vertebral body/disc ratio is less. These factors, together with the shape of the disc and amount of movement of the spine, tend to make a disc lesion more common in this region. External protrusion often creates pressure on the nerve roots giving rise to radicular pain. If the nucleus pulposus becomes internally deranged, it will give rise to the acute muscle spasm (without radicular pain) of 'lumbago'. These changes are usually gradual, occurring over a period of years, minor trauma giving only minimal physical signs or symptoms. Ultimately a relatively trivial incident causes the final trauma which produces the 'acute' disc lesion.

In the cervical region, the degeneration of age and 'wear and tear' coupled with its extreme mobility, may also cause adhesions to form between nerve roots and their sheaths. Any excessive flexion therefore, stretches the adhesions and an inflammatory state is created, giving rise to radicular pain, even without disc protrusion. In addition the normal compression force of gravity upon the discs is increased by muscle tension. This is why neck pain is often aggravated by mental tension which tends to be manifested as abnormal hypertonia in the muscles of the neck, particularly longissimus cervicis and capitis and the trapezius muscles. This increases the pressure on the discs and tends to restrict the normal blood flow.

The lumbar region is repeatedly subjected to stress, especially during forward flexion. As the discs degenerate and become less elastic they also become somewhat flattened and thinner. This creates a small amount of laxity in the capsules and ligaments of the intervertebral joints. The natural angle of inclination between L4 and L5 and at the lumbosacral junction makes them particularly liable to a shearing stress, thus increasing the 'wear and tear' on these discs. The relative 'slackness' of these joints in middle age makes them particularly liable to disc protrusion.

Acute intervertebral disc lesion

EXAMPLE

A middle-aged man tried to lift a weight which was too heavy for him, from the factory floor when in the 'stooped' position, that is, flexed with his legs straight. This resulted in right posterolateral herniation of the disc between the fourth and fifth lumbar vertebrae, which gave rise to the irritation of the right fifth lumbar nerve root. Since this root forms part of the right sciatic nerve, this will also be affected.

CLINICAL PICTURE

The patient will probably arrive at the hospital on a stretcher. Whilst his pain makes him think he cannot stand, it is unlikely to be true.

When standing it will be seen that his lumbar curve is 'flattened', which is the result of protective spasm preventing forward flexion of the lumbar spine. The erector spinae muscles on the right immediately adjacent to the lesion will be in very severe spasm causing the pelvis to be raised on the right. (See Fig. 8/1.) At about the level of L1 there is the beginning of a counter-curve to the left, making a very marked scoliosis. There may be a rotation of the lumbar vertebrae as a result of these abnormally violent muscle actions. The widespread protective spasm of the upper left lumbar muscles can be so great as to create a 'bulge' which, at first glance, may well be thought to indicate an injury in this area. This curvature is further exaggerated if forward flexion is attempted, and the left shoulder and arm will be seen to be in a line further to the left than the left hip. Tenderness is usually diffuse in the first few hours, but careful palpation will elicit an acutely tender area

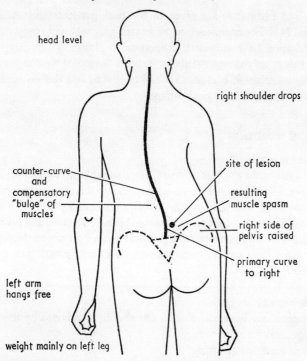

head level

right shoulder drops

site of lesion

counter-curve
and
compensatory
"bulge" of
muscles

resulting
muscle spasm

right side of
pelvis raised

primary curve
to right

left arm
hangs free

weight mainly on left leg

Fig. 8/1 Posterior view of the posture adopted by a patient with a right-sided nerve irritation from a posterolateral disc herniation, between L4 and L5.

over the lesion. Pain will be generalized in the back and radiate down the leg following the pattern of the fifth lumbar dermatome. (See also p. 216 for details of Back Examination.)

IMMEDIATE TREATMENT
Complete bed-rest is essential for the true disc protrusion. Every means to reduce the muscle spasm should be used, e.g. analgesics, ultrasound therapy and possibly even continuous traction. It is maintained until the patient has a passive pain-free straight leg-raise to 60°, which indicates a healing of the annulus.

CONSERVATIVE TREATMENT
If after bed-rest, etc., the muscle spasm is greatly reduced, then a graduated scheme of activity is introduced. Isometric exercises for

power and endurance are given to the back extensor and abdominal muscles. Mobility exercises may be started only when the signs of nerve root irritation have subsided. Sometimes a plaster corset may be applied; this is only meant to inhibit forward flexion of the lumbar spine. Therefore extension exercises should be given, and the progression is similar to that for the surgical patient.

Surgical treatment

LAMINECTOMY

If the signs and symptoms persist, after suitable investigation, it may be decided to perform a laminectomy. After this operation isometric back extension and abdominal exercises are usually started within a few days. These exercises are progressed both in duration and resistance. Whether forward flexion exercises are ever given depends on the surgeon. Many feel a fully mobile spine is essential if further back pain is to be avoided.

ADVICE TO PATIENTS

All patients who have had disc lesions should be advised by the therapist concerning the following:

correct methods of lifting;

care in activities which require sudden muscular contraction, e.g. removing a heavy object from a high shelf;

awareness of the importance of good posture in sitting, e.g. selection of a chair which fits the patient;

need for good muscle tone of both back extensor and abdominal muscles.

PROGNOSIS

This is very dependent on the patient's attitude to his injury. To many people a back injury remains a psychological barrier to activity for the rest of their lives. In fact 'backs' are one of the chief causes for work loss in this country.

For Bibliography see end of Chapter 11, p. 291.

CHAPTER 9

Major Multiple Injuries and the Physiotherapist's Approach to Athletic and Sports Injuries

M. K. PATRICK, OBE, MCSP, SRP

MAJOR MULTIPLE INJURIES

Road traffic accidents are producing many more patients with major multiple injuries. Due to the better understanding of the problems of immediate aid, more of these patients are surviving. Whilst it is estimated that 80% of the patients who sustain a traumatic rupture of the thoracic aorta die before or soon after admission to hospital, it is rare for accident patients to die of exsanguination (Porter, 1972). Whilst head and chest injuries are the major problems for the physiotherapist, the internal abdominal injuries, such as ruptures of the spleen, liver or kidneys may be of greater importance when the patient is first admitted. After the surgeon's immediate care, whatever the extent or multiplicity of the injuries that the patient has sustained, the care of the chest must be the first consideration of the physiotherapist. To enable this to be carried out efficiently, the patient's position must be changed frequently. Many trauma surgeons will carry out lengthy surgery to obtain fixation of the fractured limbs so that the patient can be turned.

Chest injury

Fractures in the chest wall can vary in severity from a fracture of one rib, which will cause little trouble in a young man, to multiple fractures of ribs leading to a completely flail chest wall, but a single broken rib in

247

a patient who has acute bronchitis is a severe complication and he may well be admitted to hospital for intensive chest physiotherapy.

Physiotherapy for patients with fractures of the chest wall can present many problems. Fractures of the ribs are very painful and it is important that the patient with even the most trivial rib fracture is given analgesics. Unless the pain is controlled the pulmonary ventilation will be decreased. This can lead to an alteration in pulmonary ventilation rate (increased speed, decreased depth of respiration). As hypercapnia may ensue, the physiotherapist must understand the significance of the measurements of blood gases as well as the techniques of chest physiotherapy. There is a natural reluctance to give any percussion to an already crushed chest and indeed it would be wrong to do so in severe injuries. To feel the fractured bone ends grinding against each other is a distressing and worrying experience to the physiotherapist who is not familiar with this type of injury. If the patient is unconscious, pain is not a problem, but this also means that the greatest care must be taken whilst treating the patient as the lung can be lacerated by the bone ends.

A patient with chest injury must have his airway kept clear and good ventilation of his lungs. How this is achieved depends on the severity of the injury and the general state of health of the patient. Most of these patients will be conscious and many will be unable or unwilling to cough. Adequate analgesics must be given to reduce the pain and in many instances it is better to arrange for this to be given in anticipation of the physiotherapist's visit. Support at the site of the fracture, by the physiotherapist's hands, will greatly help the patient to co-operate in coughing. If the patient is unable to cough a suction catheter will often stimulate the cough reflex, and the fracture site should be supported in anticipation of this coughing.

The flail chest is caused by double fractures of the same ribs, and is now very common, often caused by violent impaction with the steering-wheel of a car. Paradoxical breathing (that is, the flail section is blown out on expiration and sucked in on inspiration) is often a feature of such injuries. This paradoxical breathing has a neutralizing effect on the lung ventilation and atelectasis quickly develops. The airway must be kept clear, especially in the unconscious patient. After blood or air in the pleural cavity has been drained, some form of fixation of the flail chest is essential. This can be done by plating or wiring of the ribs so that the thorax can move normally in respiration, or by giving positive pressure ventilation through an endotracheal tube, thus ensuring that the pressure of the lung tissue supports the fractured ribs from within. It is reasonable to assume that at least ten days are required for some union of the fractured ribs to take place. The endotracheal tube can be left in situ for up to 14 days, and this would seem to be the easiest method of support. It is the most commonly used form of treatment, but it has its own complications and dangers. Cross-infection and tracheal stenosis cause a significant morbidity, if not mortality rate (Porter). Some cardio-thoracic surgeons advocate that surgical fixation of the seriously damaged chest wall should be undertaken at a relatively early stage, since pro-longed artificial ventilation is not desirable. If the clavicle is fractured as well as the upper ribs, it must be surgically reduced and fixed or a permanent deformity and limitation of chest movement will result.

The techniques that the therapist uses for these seriously ill patients are largely determined by the particular injury. It may only be possible, in the early stages, to assist the lung drainage by the position of the patient and use of the suction catheter to clear the airways. More active percussion may be necessary later. The patient will be gradually weaned off the respirator as soon as he has adequate pulmonary ventilation without assistance. (See Chapter 4 of *Chest, Heart and Vascular Disorders for Physiotherapists* for detailed physiotherapy.)

Head injury

Head injuries are now recorded at the rate of 100,000 a year. Fortunately most are relatively trivial and leave no disability. However, 60% of road accident deaths are the result of head injuries (Proctor, 1972). Of those that survive, about 1,000 a year are left with severe disablement which may be physical, intellectual, emotional or a combination of any of these. Ethically this is a very real problem to all members of the staff who are involved with these patients. Whilst the ultimate decisions are made by the medical staff, many physiotherapists are deeply concerned with their part in keeping patients alive when they have already suffered 'cerebral death'. This may have occurred as a result of the anoxia which develops when there is intracranial damage.

Initially the physiotherapist is concerned with keeping the chest functioning effectively. Often the patient is restless, even violent, when unconscious. Suitable medication helps to reduce this. Later, when the patient's level of consciousness is rising, it is often very difficult to carry out chest physiotherapy, as the patient will attempt to get out of bed or to clutch at anyone who touches him. It is usual for these patients to be nursed in an intensive therapy unit where the staff ratio is higher than in normal wards, so that nursing staff can help to control the flailing limbs and the more violent activities of the patient whilst the physiotherapist ventilates the chest. Later the patient suffers disorientation and confusion and may well be very unco-operative. Fortunately, these two stages usually pass off relatively quickly.

When the patient recovers consciousness he may be partially paralysed and unable to speak. Then follows a time when he suffers great changes of mood and frustration, and the physiotherapist, together with her colleagues, starts the often prolonged rehabilitation of the patient as a 'whole being'. Often there is so much intellectual damage that rehabilitation is greatly hampered. Regrettably, those who do overcome great physical disability are often unable to find employment. However, centres for these patients are now operating, such as that in Birmingham, and show that, given a slow introduction to the factory situation, some can re-establish their confidence and are capable of normal work. All too many head injury patients spend the rest of their lives in mental, geriatric or younger chronic sick institutions. (The detailed physiotherapy for these patients is given in Chapter VII of *Neurology for Physiotherapists.*)

Stab wounds

Stab wounds are becoming more common in many of our cities. These, too, are now so much better understood that they present less of a problem to the surgeon (Porter). To the physiotherapist they are post multiple surgery patients. Many of these stab wounds are into the chest and the principal treatment is chest ventilation.

Burns

Burns may also be a feature of multiple injuries (see Chapter 21 in *A Textbook of Medical Conditions for Physiotherapists*, 5th edition). The surgical methods of treating these has greatly reduced the scarring which was the cause of so many contractures in the past.

Whatever the extent of the injuries, chest ventilation is the first priority of the physiotherapist, and later, when survival is assured, the rest of the patient's injuries are treated by the appropriate methods.

For References and Bibliography see end of Chapter 11, page 291.

THE PHYSIOTHERAPIST'S APPROACH TO ATHLETIC AND SPORTS INJURIES

The 'athlete' has a different approach to his injury than almost any other patient who comes for physiotherapy. The injury is often a soft tissue lesion requiring similar treatment to the same lesion in a 'non-athlete', but the person is different, because for years he has devoted himself to this particular sport, often with great dedication, to the exclusion of almost everything else. His personal state of fitness is something an athlete is always aware of and strives to improve. If he stops training following an injury, he soon feels generally unwell and becomes depressed about himself and his capabilities. When he is injured he is apprehensive about his injury and the effect it will have upon his future performance. It may be easy to think of him, mistakenly, as a hypochondriac.

The athlete also has a special problem in relation to his return to his particular sport, where individual performance will be noted to the inch, or the tenth of a second of time. The footballer or cricketer returning to a team does not have this extra worry. It is possible for him to resume his sport while not at the peak of his fitness as his first appearance will be in association with other players. The mental strain is therefore less for him and it should be possible to get such a player back to his team more quickly.

Causes of injury

The injuries that these athletes and sportsmen suffer fall into two main categories, those with a known cause and those with no definite cause.

INJURIES WITH A KNOWN CAUSE

These are more obvious, because the patient has fallen or been struck by a missile, like a cricket ball. In some sports there may be a sudden violent physical contact with another player, such as occurs in football. The resultant injury is likely to recur, or at least, it is not possible for the physiotherapist to ensure that it does not do so. It is, in fact, the result of a hazard rather than a stress of sport. These are not situations which the sportsman can train himself to avoid completely. Naturally, training will include sharpening the performer's reflexes so that the injury can be minimized wherever possible. The injuries that result from these hazards of sport vary from the trivial to a major lesion.

INJURIES WITHOUT A KNOWN CAUSE

These injuries often appear to occur at a particular moment, but are really the result of a number of minor lesions which have been disregarded. Most athletes suffer some pain or discomfort whilst performing. It is often their ability to perform in spite of the pain which distinguishes the champion from the 'also ran' performer. No athlete will readily admit that he is injured and he will always hope that the pain will wear off in a few days. This means that these patients will often present themselves at a hospital when the lesion is no longer really acute. From the physiotherapist's point of view, this is a disadvantage as so often treatment given at the time of the injury would have resolved the condition, whereas a week or more after the lesion, definite changes are occurring which may be difficult to reverse.

The lesion is often due to a fault in the athlete's technique which is causing repeated minor traumata resulting in a chronic irritation of soft tissues. Muscle groups act and react in patterns of movement which normally cause no stress. If, however, the performer fails to 'carry through' the movement and performs a 'snatch-like' action, then there is considerable strain on the muscles. This is particularly true of the pain which occurs at the origin of the flexor and extensor groups of muscles in the forearm. Tennis or badminton players, javelin throwers and golfers often suffer from a chronic inflammation of the appropriate group of muscles at the elbow.

Each sport has its own pattern of movement, and therefore its own pattern of stress on the soft tissues of the body. The object of training for a sport is to build up the power and endurance of muscles so that they may perform an action repeatedly without suffering any strain. The joints must become supple but remain well controlled, if ligaments are not to be damaged. Theoretically, it would seem possible to train to a point of perfection where no stress injury could occur. In fact this is not possible, as an athlete does not train to produce a rhythmical performance. He trains to get to his 'personal best', which is a combination of technique and endurance. In competition, he will often have to force himself on to do more than the 'best' for which he has trained.

Approach to treatment

Each sport or athletic activity can provide lesions which are predictable, since they are the direct result of the pattern of stress created by the action performed. Whilst some of these are very obvious, others are not. Any physiotherapist who intends to become seriously involved in the treatment of athletic, or sports injuries, should make a careful study of the mechanics of the sport. She should also watch the sport carefully to become familiar with its hazards and to observe the mental and physical stresses of the players under competitive conditions.

All physiotherapists are well aware that they treat the patient, not the lesion. Their technique and approach has to vary with the patient's age, fitness, and mental state. It has already been stressed that the trained athlete has a particular mental approach to injury. Consequently, he needs attention paid to three aspects of his treatment: resolution of the effects of trauma; retraining in strength and endurance; and regaining of confidence in his affected limb, and its fitness for activity. When he has achieved this, he will be able to retrain for his particular sport.

Although the diagnosis will have been made before the patient is referred for treatment, the actual method of treatment used will have to be determined by the physiotherapist. In addition to the usual appraisal of the signs and symptoms, there should be a discussion with the patient as to how and when the injury occurred and which sport was involved. It may not be possible for the patient to give a particular incident as the cause of the trauma, but the athlete is so aware of his body's performance that he will know how he thinks the stress occurred.

In the first few days, the treatment will be directed primarily at resolving the acute soft tissue lesion (see Chapters 7 and 8). But the athlete's general physical state must not be ignored. Usually the injury, unless it was the result of a hazard, involves the part of the body used most in the sport and therefore normal training has to be discontinued. It follows, therefore, that a general scheme of exercises must be devised to keep the athlete in as near peak condition as possible. The best way to do this is by circuit training.

Circuit training is a familiar part of almost every athlete and sportsman's normal training schedule. It remains only for the physiotherapist to discuss with the patient what exercises his normal circuit contains and to adjust these to avoid damage to the affected area. Circuit training is a part of the normal way of life of an athlete and does not require to be performed in a hospital. Whilst the patient is having daily treatment for his acute lesion one session of circuit training can with advantage be performed there. This gives the physiotherapist the opportunity to check that the 'circuit' is safe. Later, when it is desirable to increase the muscle activity of the affected limb, the circuit is adjusted. Both the power and endurance of muscles are built up in circuit training, and so the athlete can see for himself that the injury which stopped him performing is really 'cured' and his confidence in his limb and his own ability to perform are restored.

It has been found that many athletes who have had a history of repeated small incidents of pain in a particular muscle or tendon, are very reassured if it is suggested to them, at the time of discharge from the hospital, that they might like to come for 'checks' from time to time. It is implied that it is the 'circuit' that is to be checked, but both the physiotherapist and the athlete know that this gives a reason for the athlete to return if he is worried about his old injury. This prevents a chronic state occurring, because the sportsman would be unlikely to make a formal appointment with a doctor to discuss a vague pain. The physiotherapist would of course seek medical advice for the patient if it was required. A further advantage is the prevention of more serious trauma, since it is a well-established fact that a sportsman who is unsure of his physical fitness is 'accident-prone'. His concentration is diverted to thinking about himself instead of the action he requires to make.

For References and Bibliography see end of Chapter 11, p. 292.

CHAPTER 10

Fractures

M. K. PATRICK, OBE, MCSP SRP

A fracture is a break in the continuity of bone. Most fractures occur as a result of violence.

Classification

Fractures are classified according to the pattern of the resulting bone damage. Most of the terms are self-explanatory, such as impacted (when the broken bone ends are rammed together after the fracture has occurred), and spiral or oblique (which indicate the direction of the fracture line). Some fractures involve joint surfaces or are associated with dislocations, or produce the avulsion of a piece of bone when a tendon is violently stressed.

The comminuted fracture is one in which the bone is fragmented into several pieces (see Plate 10/1, between pages 160 and 161). Children have more pliable bones and sustain greenstick fractures, which are similar to the break that would occur if a green stick were bent.

All fractures are described as simple if the skin is not broken. If the skin is broken, then they are called compound fractures. Compound or open fractures can be complicated by infection of the soft tissues or bone ends. This may occur at the time of the accident or afterwards. The skin may be broken either by an object penetrating the skin from without, or by a spike of the fractured bone protruding through it.

COMMON FRACTURES

Causes

The vast majority of fractures are sustained as a result of direct or indirect violence. It is the stresses applied to the limb at the moment of impact that determine which bone, or bones, fracture and this may not be at the point of impact.

DIRECT VIOLENCE

This may occur when a limb strikes an object and fractures. This often occurs in road accidents when the occupant of the vehicle either strikes a part of the structure of the car, or is thrown out and strikes another object.

The limb may be struck by an object as happens when a footballer is kicked and sustains a fracture.

There may be a crush injury such as a finger being caught in a closing door, or the calcanei may be crushed by jumping from a height onto one's heels.

INDIRECT VIOLENCE

A fall onto the outstretched hand accounts for most fractures of the upper arm.

Fatigue or stress fractures occur, as their name suggests, as a result of repeated stress. The 'march fracture', so called because it was frequent amongst army recruits, is the most common. It involves a fracture of the shaft or neck of the second or third metatarsal bone. Athletes who run on hard tracks or roads can sustain stress fractures of the fibula or tibia, but these are comparatively rare.

PATHOLOGICAL FRACTURES

These fractures can occur in any age-group. Whilst the fracture may occur as a result of minor trauma, the predisposition of the bone to give way under stress has been a gradual process of change in the structure of the bone, occurring over many months or even years. The patient may give a history of having stumbled and broken his leg. He attributes the fracture to the stumble, but it must be remembered that a bone with advanced changes in its structure could easily have fractured whilst the patient was asleep in bed.

The treatment for these patients will depend on the cause of the change in bone pathology. In the young it can be due to a cyst or benign tumour, but in the older age-groups it is frequently a systemic condition such as a lack of calcium ions ensuing from a nutritional or hormonal disturbance, or Paget's disease. The possibility of a malignant tumour must also be considered. If the disease is systemic, other fractures may be sustained and the physiotherapist must be very careful in the re-education programme, which should be slower than normal, as re-fracture is not uncommon.

It must always be remembered that soft tissues will be damaged in all fractures. The site of the soft tissue damage may be well away from the site of the fracture as well as immediately adjacent to it. This is particularly so in the case of indirect violence, for example a fall on the outstretched hand can result in a fracture at the wrist and damage to the soft tissue around the shoulder joint.

Signs and symptoms of fractures

Immediately after a fracture there is pain and muscle spasm. There will also be a degree of swelling and heat which varies with the way the fracture occurred and with the soft tissue damage which has been sustained. For example, if an object strikes the thigh with sufficient force to fracture the shaft of the femur, there will be a severe contusion on the aspect which was struck, plus soft tissue damage on the opposite aspect where the periosteum is torn and the bone ends project into the muscles. The thigh muscles are very vascular and so the resulting haematoma will be considerable and the area will be hot as well as swollen.

If, however, the fracture is an undisplaced one of the scaphoid, caused by falling on an outstretched hand, whilst there will be pain and tenderness at the fracture site, there will be minimal, if any, visible swelling. The soft tissue contusion on the palm of the hand, where it struck the ground, would not normally be great, and the haemorrhage from the bone would be slight and contained within the periosteum.

Displacement, causing alteration in body contours, or the position or attitude of limbs, can be a very marked sign of a fracture. It is confirmed by X-ray evidence. When there is a fracture the bone ends must move, but they can return to their original position (undisplaced fracture), or be driven into each other (impacted fracture). More usually they are displaced. The degree of displacement depends on the number of muscles and their power and direction of pull on the bone fragments, as well as the degree and direction of the stress which caused the fracture. Usually this displacement has to be reduced in order to obtain normal, or as near normal as possible, re-alignment of the fragments. This is done because union will only occur if the fragments are in apposition and the limb can only be functional again if its architecture is correct. It must also be remembered that whilst jagged bone ends are protruding into soft tissues they can cause further damage, either by pressure or by laceration. This extra damage could involve not only the muscles, but blood vessels and nerves. It is for this reason that even the most seriously injured patient will have his fracture reduced as soon as the essential life-saving procedures have been carried out. Only when the fractures are securely held can the nursing and physiotherapy procedures needed by these patients be given safely and adequately.

Repair

The repair of the bone is similar to the repair of other connective tissues. It differs only in the activity of specialized cells which lay down new bone, and in the calcification of the matrix. The specialized bone-forming cells are derived from the periosteum and endosteum of the damaged area. Some reticulo-endothelial cells from the bone marrow also seem to have the ability to take on an osteogenic function. The type of activity of all these cells depends on the stimulus which is provided. Too much movement at the fracture site stimulates the production of fibrous tissue. For bone to be laid down, the fracture area must be relatively immobile.

STAGES OF FRACTURE REPAIR

The stages of fracture repair which will be considered are: (*i*) haematoma formation and organization; (*ii*) subperiosteal proliferation, procallus; (*iii*) callus formation, woven bone; (*iv*) consolidation, lamellar bone; and (*v*) remodelling.

It should be remembered that these stages fuse with each other, and that more than one stage may be going on at the same time in different parts of the fracture site.

HAEMATOMA FORMATION AND ORGANIZATION

Bone is a highly vascular tissue. When cortical bone is broken, the vessels of the Haversian systems are ruptured, and a few millimetres of ischaemic bone will therefore die. This dead bone is gradually absorbed over a few days, leaving a gap between the cortical bone ends. Cancellous bone has a more open meshwork, and less necrosis occurs.

Between both types of bone, profuse bleeding occurs at the time of fracture, and a haematoma will form, which is usually contained by the periosteum. The haematoma forms the basis for the type of repair which would occur in any wound. New capillaries penetrate the haematoma, fibres are laid down and granulation tissue is thus formed. This should be regarded as a temporary repair process as the granulation tissue does not form the basis of the true bony repair.

SUBPERIOSTEAL PROLIFERATION—PROCALLUS

Simultaneously with the formation of granulation tissue (by the second or third day after the fracture), there is proliferation of cells in the area immediately adjacent to the damaged periosteum and endosteum. These cells may lay down primitive bone, or occasionally, small areas of cartilage. The combination of the subperiosteal collar thus formed and the soft granulation tissue makes a weak link between the broken bone ends. This is known as provisional callus, or procallus.

It is essential that the fracture site is protected from major stress at this time. The body is capable of this without assistance, by the interaction of the pain/muscle spasm cycle. Muscle spasm keeps the bone ends together until healing has occurred, and provided that there is good bony alignment, a reasonable result will be obtained. However, the certainty of good repair and maintained alignment, with pain relief, can be better obtained by the use of artificial aids such as plaster casts or internal fixation (see page 262).

CALLUS FORMATION—WOVEN BONE

The area of activity of the cells which formed the subperiosteal collar gradually extends. Provided that the fracture site is kept relatively immobile, the cells lay down an osteoid material in a calcified matrix. The osteoid trabeculae show no particular pattern, hence the term 'woven bone'. When the woven bone extends between the bone ends and thus bridges the fracture site, it is visible on X-ray. This does not mean that the repair is strong enough to withstand the stress of weight-bearing or heavy activity, or that the woven bone extends fully through the area previously occupied by the haematoma. It will take time for this to occur. The granulation tissue is absorbed as the woven bone extends.

CONSOLIDATION—LAMELLAR BONE

The simultaneous activity of osteoblasts and osteoclasts gradually replaces the woven bone with lamellar bone. This is the type of bone which will withstand the strains and stresses of weight-bearing. The trabecular pattern is similar to that found in normal bone and has a 'ply' arrangement. When lamellar bone has been formed, full bony union is said to have occurred, and the fracture repair is complete.

REMODELLING

Although lamellar bone is strong, the appearance of the bone may be far from normal. Excess bone may be present at the fracture site, or the bone ends may have healed without perfect alignment. These imperfections are gradually adjusted, as the bone is constantly remodelled by continuous osteoblast and osteoclast activity.

GENERAL PRINCIPLES OF TREATMENT

Basically, all treatment is performed hoping for a complete recovery to normal function. It is the surgeon's hope that he can obtain and maintain perfect alignment of the fractured bone ends. The physiotherapist hopes for full range and power. Often the results that have to be accepted are less than this, not because of the failure or lack of skill, but because the two aims are not always compatible. It is, therefore, worth considering what is acceptable, and why.

UPPER LIMB

This is a non-weight-bearing limb, which needs range of movement and dexterity. Neither of these are of use if the nerve supply to the hand is absent, for the arm moves to allow the hand to act.

Some degree of loss of length of bones or deformity can be accepted, as long as the retained range is functionally useful. If immobilized for more than two or three weeks, both the shoulder and the elbow will develop soft tissue changes which result in permanent loss of range. In the over-60 age-group, these changes occur in a week, if there is soft tissue damage to the joint. Therefore, early movement takes precedence over the need for good bone alignment. The early rehabilitation programme is planned for range of movement and followed by a power-building programme.

LOWER LIMB

This is a weight-bearing limb. Any shortening or deformity which occurs will affect the gait and posture of the patient. Therefore, every effort is made to obtain and maintain correct bone alignment whilst union is taking place. In order to achieve this, it may be necessary to immobilize the limb in plaster for many months, and perhaps to adopt more than one procedure of treatment (e.g. a bone graft, or plating operation when union has failed to take place after the limb has been in plaster for several months). Long periods of immobilization may well result in some permanent loss of joint range.

The primary aim of the rehabilitation programme after lower limb injury is controlled movement, since stability is of the greatest importance. The patient will soon learn to accommodate to any loss of joint range. A patient may have an arthrodesed hip or knee joint and is able to regain functional activity; but a patient who has a knee joint that does not fully extend is at a great disadvantage because the quadriceps cannot work efficiently.

In the ankle joint, loss of dorsiflexion can be accommodated by raising the heel of the shoe, or loss of plantarflexion may be overcome by shortening the stride. The subtalar joint is usually painful if its range is not full. This patient finds himself unable to walk on any surface, other than a perfectly flat one, without great pain, and this may well be so intolerable that the joint has to be arthrodesed. This operation, whilst relieving the pain, leaves the patient with a severe disability, and such an altered gait pattern that a very careful and often prolonged rehabilitation programme has to be undertaken.

SUPPORTS FOR FRACTURES

These are not always necessary, but if they are used, they can be applied either externally or internally.

External

LARGE ARM SLINGS

Impacted fractures of the upper limb are often rested in a large arm sling. This may well be worn under the clothes for the first few days, but should not be retained there for longer than seven to ten days, because the shoulder joint, especially in the elderly, soon loses its range of movement.

The 'collar and cuff' is designed to provide a slight traction (the weight of the arm) on the shoulder joint whilst restricting the movement of the joint.

STRAPPING, ETC

Some fractures do not require reduction. For example, fractures of the outer toes will unite spontaneously. They are seldom grossly displaced and the tendons will support the fractures. They do not require any further support, but sometimes a collodion bandage is applied, more for the reasurance of the patient than any other reason. Fractures of the shaft of the middle phalanges of the fingers are similarly supported by the tendons. It is usual to apply two narrow bands of strapping, one distal and one proximal to the fracture, enclosing the finger next to the one injured, which is thus used for support.

Fractures of the distal phalanx are often displaced because of the muscular attachments. These are usually supported on the palmar aspect, on a small ($1\frac{1}{2}$ inches, 38 mm) gutter splint which is held in position by strapping. The advantage of this light support is that functional use of the limb can be resumed at once.

PLASTER CASTS

The majority of fractures are reduced and supported in a plaster cast. This cast is not meant to hold the fractured bone ends rigid. It would be impossible for the cast to do so because of the bulk of soft tissues between it and the bone. It is meant to support the limb and prevent gross displacement recurring as a result of severe muscle spasm or external force.

In order to give greater stability to the fracture the joints adjacent to it may be included. Indeed, it is said that the joints immediately above and below should be included, but frequently one of these may be excluded. For example, a forearm plaster for a Colles fracture does not normally include the elbow joint. If the elbow joint is not immobilized, some pronation and supination can take place. However, an elbow joint soon stiffens when it is immobilized. This could produce a major disability following a relatively trivial injury of the wrist which did not require perfect alignment for functional use.

The lower limb function is weight-bearing, and therefore good anatomical alignment is essential. For this reason, it is usual to treat severe fractures of the lower leg in a long plaster (groin to base of toes). This is retained at least until some union has taken place, then the knee joint may be freed so that it can be mobilized.

THOMAS'S SPLINTS, ETC.

It is sometimes necessary to give prolonged traction to a fracture, to reduce the overlapping bone ends and then to maintain them in apposition. For this technique, there are several types of frame. These splints can either be designed for the support of injuries to the upper leg, in which case they are full-length, and based on the principle of the Thomas's splint, or they are modified for the treatment of the lower leg, Braun's splints.

Internal Fixation

This term is used to describe the fixation of a fracture by an operative procedure in which a metal support is used. This may be a medullary nail, which is within the bone; or a plate, screws or wire bands applied to the bone. Some surgeons will not use internal fixation unless other non-operative procedures have failed, or there is some other overriding reason. This is because of the hazards of the technique (e.g. bone sepsis, tissue/metal reactions, fatigue fractures of the metal, etc.). However, in recent years, many of the problems associated with internal fixation have been better understood, and overcome. The advocates of the Swiss A.O. technique of compression plating (Arbeitgemeinschaft für Osteosynthesefragen, see page 265) feel that compression is essential for the success of internal fixation.

ADVANTAGES OF INTERNAL FIXATION

Fractures with severe displacement may be very difficult to reduce without an open operation. To maintain the corrected position prolonged traction may be required, or it may be quite impossible without an operation and internal fixation. Unless the broken bone ends are kept in close proximity to each other no bony union can take place. The fixation does not of itself speed up the repair processes, but it does make it possible.

Another reason for internal fixation can be the desire to mobilize the patient quickly. This is especially true of the elderly patient with a fractured neck of femur, who could well become a chronic invalid if he were required to stay in bed for twelve weeks whilst his fracture united.

The Smith-Petersen pin for the fractured neck of femur was one of the first means of internal fixation to be universally adopted. A few weeks after the operation the patient was able to walk in a weight-relieving caliper. Over the years a great deal of progress has been made in improving operation techniques, and new metals have become available, so that today there are many different types of nails, pins, plates, screws and prostheses available to the surgeon as methods of internal fixation for many types of fracture.

PLATING
If a plate is applied at once, there is a danger that a 'gap' might be created between the bone ends as reabsorption takes place. If this 'gap' becomes too wide, the periosteal and endosteal bone-forming cells (osteoblasts) will not be activated, and a fibrous union will be formed. For this reason, plating is usually delayed.

No plate, pin or screw is designed to take full weight-bearing until it is supported by a bony union. The purpose of the fixation is to try to maintain the proximity of the bone ends. After most of these operations, a plaster cast, or other support, is still required. In medullary nailing and A.O. compression plating, the limb is free for non-weight-bearing exercise.

MEDULLARY NAILS
The use of nails inserted into the medullary cavity to support fractures, especially spiral or comminuted fractures, was described by Rush in 1955 (see Plate 11/2 between pages 160 and 161). These are often used in fractures of the humeral shaft, since they allow for careful early movement of the shoulder joint. Rarely they are used for fractures of the femoral shaft, since they are not sufficiently rigid in the fixation. However, they are used in pairs, in tibial fractures, especially as a delayed procedure for fractures that do not seem to be uniting. A supporting plaster is usually applied.

Küntscher advocated a much stouter nail which gave greater rigidity. These are often used for middle-third fractures of the femur, especially if the patient is of slight build, because weight-bearing can be started as soon as the surgeon feels there is a bridging callus formation. There is a tendency for these patients, who are quite pain-free, to feel that the leg is normal and subject it to too much stress. Some surgeons, therefore, keep their patients on sticks longer than they appear to need them. Certainly, a small proportion of the patients who have these nails inserted have non-union, or refracture a few months later. This is thought by some to be due to the damage to the medullary circulation caused by the nail. The physiotherapist should watch for any loss of joint range or complaint of pain, as this is often a sign that excessive stress is being put upon the fracture site and that malunion is occurring.

INTERNAL FIXATION WITH COMPRESSION (See Fig. 10/1)
In the Swiss A.O. method of fixation with compression, the operative procedure aims at an accurate alignment of the bone fragments with a

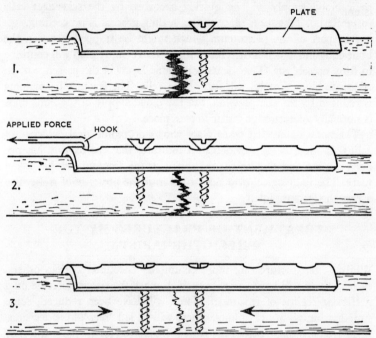

Fig. 10/1 Compression plating. 1. The first hole is drilled approximately 1 cm from the fracture. The plate is applied and the screw inserted so that the head just touches the plate. 2. The fracture is then reduced accurately and the compression force applied. The second hole is drilled as far as possible from the fracture site through the next hole in the plate. 3. Pressure of the head of each of these screws against the flange of the hole will further compress the fractured fragments. (Further screws are then inserted into the remaining holes.)

rigid fixation of the fracture, at the same time preserving the vitality of the soft tissues and bone. A few days after the operation, the patient is pain-free, and the limb has no external support, so that non-weight-bearing exercises can be started at once.

REPAIR OF BONE

When internal fixation with compression is used, there is a different process of repair, since there is no movement, and no space between the bone fragments. If the fixation is rigid so that shearing and torsional forces cannot act, no major reabsorption of the bone ends takes place. However, any minute bone fragments or spicules which are denuded of their blood supply will be quickly absorbed by the scavenger cells (osteoclasts). This takes place as the healing process is proceeding.

Any part of the periosteum which might be trapped between the bone ends and which is therefore subjected to compression will continue to form osteoblasts. That is, its osteogenic layer, in the presence of an adequate blood supply, will form bone cells. The fracture haematoma is reduced by the compression, but the blood supply of the bone ends is normally adequate for repair to take place.

The bony union that takes place shows no radiological evidence of callus. If there is such evidence, it indicates that the fixation has not been perfect and that some movement at the fracture site has taken place. The radiological evidence of union is the presence of trabeculae across the fracture line.

TREATMENT OF FRACTURES BY THE PHYSIOTHERAPIST

Whilst some fractures are more commonly encountered than others, each of these will have variations which make the surgeon decide on a particular regime of treatment. Some will have been reduced, some supported in plaster or splints, others will be left free. These decisions will have been made before the patient is referred for therapy, and they will affect the treatment only in detail.

It is important to remember why the fracture is being treated. It is not to obtain perfect bone alignment which looks excellent on X-ray. It is to restore to the limb as full a function as possible. Often a compromise has to be reached and the best alignment that can be achieved without the risk of permanently affecting the range of movement of an adjacent joint has to be accepted.

Fractures that do not require major support

Many of these fractures are of minor bones, or of ones which would lead to joint stiffness if immobilized.

Fractures

A fracture remains a fracture until it is fully united, whether it is supported in a plaster cast or left free, and the physiotherapist must select suitable activity, at each stage. For example, a patient with a fractured metacarpal can reasonably be expected to try to grip a small ball on the day after his injury, but not be asked to carry and stack bricks. An elderly patient with an impacted fracture of the neck of the humerus, will require assistance when asked to raise his arm in the early stages of rehabilitation.

It is important to apply common sense, as well as professional expertise, as to the choice of activity. The degree of functional activity normal for the patient is the aim. By talking to the patient about his hobbies, mode of living, and work, the physiotherapist can ascertain the patient's normal use of his affected limb. The young man with fractured metacarpals, who is a bricklayer, will need a different type of hand movement and muscle power, which may be comparatively weak. It is mobility which he needs, and which he is likely to lose quickly and permanently if the rehabilitation programme is not planned properly.

Fractures in plaster

When a patient with a fracture in plaster is referred to the physiotherapist for treatment, the rehabilitation programme should include: maintenance of mobility of all joints which are not enclosed in plaster; and isometric exercises for all muscle groups enclosed in the plaster.

After the plaster is removed, the gaining of lost joint movement and muscle power are the primary aims of treatment. It is in the first few days of this section of the rehabilitation programme that the physiotherapist must watch for signs of non-union. This shows as swelling, heat and tenderness and even reddening of the skin over the fractured area, indicating an acute inflammatory state. Normally a patient will attempt to move stiffened joints and resume normal function of the affected area with encouragement. If he does not, it is often a sign that union is not quite complete. During the first week after the plaster has been removed there is no long-term advantage in 'forcing on' with activity, rather it should be an attempt to get the patient to start using the limb normally, and once this is achieved mobility and strength quickly return.

Fractures of the lower limb treated by prolonged traction
(e.g. Thomas's splints)

The amount of exercise that can be given is limited by the fixation. If skin traction to the lower leg is the method used, then foot and ankle movements are given with especial care to watch for any paralysis due to pressure on the peroneal nerve, and for pressure sores over the tendo achilles. Knee movements are often very delayed in this fixed traction technique and it is seldom used today. The disadvantage of the prolonged traction method is the stiffness of the knee, which may take as long as two years to recover full range.

More usually a Steinmann's pin is inserted through the tibial condyles and sliding traction is given by means of a stirrup. Foot and ankle movements and isometric contractions are given at once. Knee flexion, within the confines of the splint, are permitted as soon as clinical union has taken place.

A Braun frame is seldom used in this country for the treatment of fractures of the femur. However, it is used for fractures of the tibia, especially those which have had open surgery. It is used more as a resting splint than as a means of applying traction. The amount of physiotherapy that is given depends on the particular fracture being treated and on the method used.

Fractures treated by internal fixation

Early activity is nearly always requested for patients who have had internal fixation applied. It must be remembered that no weight-bearing or resistance that could cause a strain on the plate, screws or pins is given until bony union is established.

Smith-Petersen pins and other devices to stabilize hip fractures, medullary nails and A.O. compression plates are all used to allow immediate freedom of movement. The exercises chosen are in keeping with the fracture and the musculature of the patient. The frail elderly patient who has had a hip fracture may need help to lift her leg for the first few days, whereas the young fit man should have sufficient muscle power to perform this action.

When plating (non-compression) is used, the limb is usually enclosed in a plaster cast until clinical union has taken place. These patients are given exercises as for any other patient in plaster.

Compression plating and screwing by the A.O. method allows immediate free movement of the limb. Even if the fracture goes into a joint, active movements should be given immediately. The limb is elevated for the first few days. A tibial fracture is often rested on a Braun's frame to allow the initial inflammation to subside. Localized treatment for this is seldom needed as the generalized activity of the limb enables the inflammation to resolve spontaneously and quickly.

This A.O. method of treating fractures of the tibia enables the patient to have full joint movement at all times. There is a special caliper that is used to allow early walking whilst preventing weight-bearing on the fracture site (see Plate 10/2).

Once weight-bearing is allowed some care should be taken for the first few days. It must be remembered that the patient has been in no pain for some weeks and feels able to do everything. There will be no evidence of callus on the X-ray. It is the presence of trabeculae across the 'old fracture line' that will determine whether union has been consolidated, plus the absence of pain on 'springing' the fracture, or on palpation. The physiotherapist should watch the fracture area carefully for the first signs of non-union, that is, the *first* sign of swelling, redness or tenderness and note the most casual remark about pain. To wait and see 'how it is tomorrow' can be too late, as 24 hours of activity can loosen the metal fixation. It is essential to report these signs at once to the surgeon. It is better to be proved incorrect in one's suspicions than to miss an ununited fracture. This is of course true of all fractures, not only those which have metal implants.

Disability of a fracture

It is always important to remember that a limb in plaster makes normal living more difficult, and sometimes impossible. A frail elderly patient with a wrist in plaster may be living alone. She may be unable to undress or dress herself. Even moving a kettle of boiling water may be too heavy for her with one hand. Care must be taken to ensure that neighbours are asked to help, or the patient will soon show signs of debility from malnutrition and lack of personal care.

No elderly patient should ever be sent home non-weight-bearing on crutches or a frame, unless the home circumstances have been investigated to ensure that someone will call regularly to see that the patient is able to cope and has not fallen. It is worth remembering that many old people interpret 'non-weight-bearing' as meaning that they are simply not to walk on the limb. The writer has known many patients with hip fractures who thought doing housework on their knee was non-weight-bearing!

Progression of treatment

This depends principally on the age of the patient. The elderly must be encouraged to keep their joints moving and, as far as the injury will allow, to keep 'on their feet'. Even a few weeks of bed-rest will be disabling to them.

Children on the other hand will regain joint range and power with very little help, and even severe fractures with poor alignment will be remodelled, surprisingly well, in time. Young children should not normally be given regular treatment in a physiotherapy department. It is better to reassure and advise the parent and let the child make its own progress, with 'checks' at intervals. The biggest deterrent to this progress is an over-anxious parent, and at the 'check' visits it is often the parent who needs reassurance, rather than the child who needs physiotherapy.

Long-term care

When the patient has reasonable functional use of the limb and is confident in his ability, regular physiotherapy should be discontinued. The long-term recovery often takes many months, even a year for a major fracture. At this stage, the patient should be encouraged to take responsibility for his further progress. Normal use in daily living is all that should be needed to restore the part to full function. 'Check' appointments should be given so that the physiotherapist can be sure that progress is being made. Should it be found that the patient is losing range or power, an investigation as to the cause should be made, and perhaps a short, intensive course of treatment given.

For Bibliography see end of Chapter 11, p. 292.

CHAPTER 11

Charts of Common Fractures

M. K. PATRICK, OBE, MCSP, SRP

The following is a précis of the more common fractures that the physiotherapist can expect to see. When referring to this section, it is important to recall the previous detail that has been presented in the earlier chapters. For example, soft tissue damage will have occurred at the time of the fracture and may well influence the physiotherapy that is given, both in the early and late stages of rehabilitation.

Points to bear in mind when reading the charts

COLUMN 1
It is impossible to describe a typical fracture. The variations that can occur are legion.

COLUMN 2 USUAL AGE-GROUP
This is, as it says, an indication of the age-group which most frequently sustains this type of fracture. It must be remembered that almost any fracture can be sustained by a person of any age.

COLUMN 3 HOW INJURY OCCURS
This suggests the most usual but by no means the only way to sustain the fracture.

COLUMN 4 MOST USUAL METHOD OF FIXATION
The surgeon will consider many factors before selecting his method of treatment. Whilst an internal fixation with a plate might be the choice for an adult, it would be unsuitable for a child, whose bones are still

271

growing. One or two more common methods have been listed here for the guidance of the physiotherapist.

COLUMN 5 MOVEMENTS BEGUN
This is, of necessity, only a guide to the timing of progression. The surgeon will indicate his requirements, which will be based on local factors such as the general health of the patient, the degree of stability of the fracture, etc. The terms 'weight-bearing' and 'non-weight-bearing in plaster' indicate the time at which some weight can be expected to be taken on the limb.

In the charts and notes which follow, some broad outlines of treatment are given, and the reasons for them. It must be remembered that all injuries are different, as are the people that sustain them. The treatment must be given to meet the needs of the particular patient, *not* as they appear in any book.

COMMON FRACTURES—(TRAUMATIC)

Fractures of the shoulder region	Usual age-group	How injury occurs	Most usual method of fixation	Movements begun	Complications	Results and comments
CLAVICLE —Outer third	Any	Fall on outstretched hand	1. Sling for a few days or 2. 'Figure of 8' bandages	Immediately	—	Excellent. Large callus diminishes with time
SCAPULA —Glenoid —Neck —Acromion —Body	Adult	Direct blow or crush	Sling for a few days	Immediately	—	Excellent. Usually unites with fibrous tissue but this is not detrimental to function
HUMERUS— —Gt Tuberosity				Immediately	—	Excellent in the younger age-groups
—Gt Tuberosity with dislocation of shoulder	Adult	Fall on outstretched hand	Sling for a few days	After 24 hours	Axillary nerve lesion	The elderly nearly always lose range of shoulder movement
—Surgical neck (impacted) See Plate 11/1	Elderly	Fall on outstretched hand	1. Sling for a few days	Immediately	—	Results vary. If the impaction leaves a poor bony architecture range may be very limited
—Shaft	Adult	Direct blow	1. Operation. Rush nail and sling 3 weeks or 2. Guarding plaster 4–6 weeks	Immediately, avoiding rotation As soon as practicable	Radial nerve or blood vessel damage	Good Stiff elbow and shoulder if patient is elderly

Notes

RANGE

Normally an arm can move through an arc of 360°. This requires free movement of the shoulder joint and the shoulder girdle. With age this range becomes slightly diminished. After injury it is very important to prevent further loss of this range, for it is difficult, if not impossible, to regain. Immediate, carefully assisted movements are therefore given whenever possible.

Loss of range will reduce the functional use of the whole limb.

POWER

Full power can only be restored if the range is full. The easiest and safest way to restore power is by normal usage.

COMPLICATIONS

Immediately after injury the only way a nerve lesion can be detected is by loss or alteration in skin sensation. Blood vessel damage is observed as discoloration and swelling of fingers and hand. Test by pinching tips of the fingers and observing speed of blood return.

FRACTURED CLAVICLE

This can be treated with a 'figure of 8' bandage; this does not support the fracture. It can cause great discomfort in the axillae. It is used less often now. This fracture, if combined with a 'flail' chest lesion, is serious.

FRACTURE DISLOCATION OF SHOULDER

This is a common injury in the elderly. Range must be maintained. This can be done if great care is taken to support the weight of the limb when the patient is performing movements. Axillary nerve lesion is fairly common. It is not always easy to see whether deltoid muscle is working for several weeks, but the skin sensation of the C5 nerve will be altered. If the nerve is involved the need for maintaining the range of movement is still of the greatest importance. In most instances there is spontaneous recovery from the nerve compression.

FRACTURED SHAFT OF HUMERUS

Blood vessel damage is not common. If it occurs it is usually noted in the casualty department and dealt with there. Loss of extension of the wrist may not be observed for a day or two after injury (radial nerve lesion).

COMMON FRACTURES—(TRAUMATIC)

Fractures of the elbow region	Usual age-group	How injury occurs	Most usual method of fixation	Movements begun	Complications	Results and comments
SUPRA-CONDYLAR	Child	Fall	1. Collar and cuff 3 weeks *or* 2. Guarding plaster axilla to wrist 3 weeks	Encourage all possible movements immediately	Blood vessel or nerve lesion	Perfect in time, may take a year if damage has been severe
RADIUS —Head (undisplaced)	Any	Fall on outstretched hand	1. Sling for a few days	Immediately		Full recovery
—Head (with more than a third of articular surface involved)	Adult		1. Operation. Excision and sling 7–10 days	Immediately gentle flexion/extension		90% of range recovered in middle-aged 75% of range recovered in the elderly
—Neck			1. Sling for a few days	Immediately	Radial nerve lesion (rare)	Good results
ULNA —Olecranon	Any	Forced flexion of the elbow	1. Operation. Lag screw (compression) or wired and sling 3 weeks *or*	Elbow movements at 2–4 weeks (earlier for elderly patients)	Ulnar nerve lesion. Medial nerve lesion (very rare)	Some loss of range. This often returns, after use, over a period of months
			2. 3–4 weeks guarding plaster	Elbow movements when plaster removed		Poor, now seldom used because of joint stiffness for adults
—Monteggia's (fracture dislocation of ulna and dislocation of radius) *See Plate 11/2*	Adult	Direct blow (e.g. road traffic accident). Forced pronation	1. Operation. Plated or nailed and wired. Screwed and sling 2 weeks *or*	Elbow movements at 2–3 weeks		Results depend on post-reduction bone architecture
			2. Axilla to metacarpal joint plaster 4–5 weeks	Elbow movements when plaster removed		Poor, now seldom used because of joint stiffness for adults. Used for children

RANGE

Forearm rotation (pro- and supination). The functional usefulness of the hand after an elbow injury is proportional to the degree of rotation regained. It is re-educated in functional activity only.

Flexion. The hand must reach the mouth, beyond this flexion is not essential.

Extension. Whilst full range movements are always the aim, an arm with no extension beyond 90° can be functional, if the other movements are good.

Never attempt to increase the range by passive movements.

POWER

Active use is the only safe way to increase the muscle power of an elbow. Any attempt to 'hurry' the recovery by weight-lifting, etc., will invariably result in loss of range and muscle spasm.

COMPLICATIONS

Blood vessel damage. Whilst this is rare, it is extremely important to watch for signs in the first few days. A dead-white hand and forearm which is acutely tender must be reported at once. It could be a sign of Volkmann's ischaemia, which if dealt with immediately is reversible, but if delayed can result in permanent paralysis.

A discoloured, swollen hand (venous congestion) must also be reported. It is usually caused by the plaster being too tight, or the deformity of the limb impeding the venous return.

SOFT TISSUE DAMAGE

In elbow injuries this is often extensive, resulting in considerable swelling. In adults it tends to organize and give rise to permanent limitation of joint movements if it is not treated. Fortunately few elbow injuries of adults need to be in plaster, so that ultrasound therapy can be given at once, even if movement is not permitted. Children are treated in plaster, since operative procedures are avoided, but the stiffness resulting from the soft tissue damage is soon freed, once movement is allowed.

SUPRACONDYLAR FRACTURES

Either or both condyles can be fractured, causing considerable derangement of the joint. This is primarily an injury of children, who are treated in a guarding plaster. Swelling is considerable and a close watch must be kept to see that venous congestion does not occur and that the fingers are kept fully mobile. The immediate results are often not good but the bony architecture is improved in the later stages of bone repair and the range of movements improves as the deformity lessens.

FRACTURE OF HEAD OR NECK OF RADIUS

Early movement is essential for good results.

FRACTURED OLECRANON AND MONTEGGIA'S FRACTURE

In order to maintain the postoperative position movements cannot be given at once. When they are permitted remember to use triceps only 'smoothly' and gently until bony union has taken place, or the olecranon may be pulled off again.

COMMON FRACTURES—(TRAUMATIC)

Fractures of forearm	Usual age-group	How injury occurs	Most usual method of fixation	Movements begun	Complications	Results and comments
ULNA —Shaft	Any	Direct blow	1. Compression plating 3 weeks *or*	Immediate gentle flexion and extension of elbow		Fairly good. Some loss of forearm rotation
			2. Plating and forearm plaster 4 to 6 weeks *or*	Flexion and extension of elbow 1 to 3 weeks	Non-union	
			3. Axilla to metacarpophalangeal joint long plaster 6–8 weeks	Flexion and extension of elbow when plaster removed		Poor, considerable loss of forearm rotation and some loss of flexion/extension of elbow. Improves over years in children. Seldom used for adults
RADIUS AND ULNA —Shafts	Any	Direct blow or fall	1. Compression plate to *each* bone and sling 4 weeks *or*	Immediately gentle flexion and extension of elbow	Non-union especially of ulna	Good results
			2. Plating of one or both bones and plaster 4–6 weeks *or*	Immediately plaster removed gentle flexion and extension of elbow	Non-union especially of ulna	Fairly good if both bones are plated, some loss of forearm rotation
			3. Axilla to metacarpal joint plaster 6–12 weeks		Cross-union	Poor, considerable loss of forearm rotation and flexion/extension. Improves over the years with children. Seldom used for adults

Notes

RANGE

Flexion and extension of the elbow and wrist are not affected unless the limb is put into a long plaster. Usually only children are treated in plaster, since operative procedures are avoided. These joints mobilise quite quickly.

An adult would lose elbow range permanently if kept in plaster for any length of time.

Forearm rotations. These cannot be permitted until some bony union has taken place. Rotations must be re-educated with *great* care, or non-union or a re-fracture will occur. Usually these movements are only given as part of a functional action.

POWER

This is quickly regained once *firm* union is established. The overall time for complete rehabilitation is often shortened if 'strengthening exercises' for the arm are delayed. The power of the hand in a 'gripping' action should be encouraged from the beginning.

COMPLICATIONS

Blood vessels and nerves are sometimes damaged at the same time since these fractures are usually the result of direct blows and often occur in road traffic accidents. However, they are not complications in the normal sense of the word, in that they do not occur as a result of the fracture.

Non-union is the most likely complication, particularly of the ulna, which is slow to unite and forms only a fibrous union. Heat, swelling or tenderness over the fracture area or pain or sudden loss of forearm rotation should be regarded as possible indications of non-union or re-fracture.

PHYSIOTHERAPY

This must be directed towards encouraging use rather than attempting to 'hurry' recovery. These injuries are difficult to treat. Delayed movements seem to be adding to the overall joint stiffness, yet any attempt to force movements always meets with disaster.

COMMON FRACTURES—(TRAUMATIC)

Fractures of the wrist and hand	Usual age-group	How injury occurs	Most usual method of fixation	Movements begun	Complications	Results and comments
RADIUS —lower end— Colles' (See Plate 11/3) —Smith's	Over-50	Fall on outstretched hand Blow on back of wrist	Short plaster 4–6 weeks (Colles' plaster) i.e. below elbow to knuckles with thumb free	Use in plaster. Once plaster is removed all movements are given	Rupture of extensor pollicis longus. Causalgia (median nerve compression). Sudek's atrophy	Good function, but often considerable deformity. Contours improve with time
SCAPHOID	Young adult males	Fall on outstretched hand	'Scaphoid' plaster 4–12 weeks (i.e. below elbow to knuckles with carpo-metacarpal joint of thumb enclosed)	Use in plaster. Once plaster is removed all movements given	Non-union. Necrosis, usually result of fracture not being immobilized immediately	90% unite, good results
METACARPALS	Young males	Direct blow (boxing)	1. None or strapping for a few days or 2. Colles' plaster 3 weeks	Immediately full use. Exercises		Loss of knuckles. Full function
BENNETT'S (1st metacarpal) (See Plate 11/4)	Any	Direct blow	1. None or strapping for a few days or 2. Operation, screwed	Immediately exercises Exercises after 10 days		Risk of stiffness from plaster is too great in elderly. Therefore immediate use is usually ordered

PHALANGES	Any	Direct blow Rotational strain	Girdle strapping 10–14 days (affected finger to next)	Immediately Normal use of hand	Function excellent. If articular surface is involved there will always be loss of joint range, which seldom impairs function

Notes

FUNCTION

Power and pincer-type grips are the primary functions of the hand. In order to perform these actions effectively, normal kinaesthetic sensation, good joint range and controlled muscle power are needed

RANGE

The joints of the wrist and hand are a complex structure designed to perform very strong and very delicate movements. The actual range of movement of each joint varies with the individual, and comparison with the uninjured hand is the only guide to their normal range.

Since function is the essential feature of the hand, it is this, rather than particular joint range, which should be the aim. Shoulder movements should be carefully checked.

POWER

This is very important in the hand. All re-education should be designed towards power. Joint range is of no benefit if it is not controlled by strong muscle power.

COSMETIC APPEARANCE

This is often sacrificed in order to keep the functional range, e.g. fractured metacarpals usually result in the 'loss' of a knuckle because of a slight overlapping of the bone ends. To obtain a cosmetically perfect result would require an operative procedure which could result in a loss of metacarpophalangeal joint range.

COLLES' AND SMITH'S FRACTURES

A post-reduction 'slipping' of the bones often leads to a deformity, but this seldom interferes with function.

COMPLICATIONS

Late rupture of E.P.L. This is fairly common with elderly patients. It may happen at three weeks or three months after injury.

Causalgia. This is rare, and is caused by compression of median nerve. Symptoms: hypersensitivity and exquisite pain, mainly over thenar eminence.

Sudek's atrophy. This is only seen in patients who are fearfully unable or unwilling to use the hand. Clinically the hand is shiny, reddish in colour and swollen. X-rays show osteoporosis. It is almost impossible to regain movements if this syndrome has really become established, as this patient will not co-operate. It must be anticipated and prevented.

Persistent wrist pain (weeks after union) may be due to subluxation of radio-ulnar joint. Excision of distal portion of ulna may be necessary.

SCAPHOID FRACTURE

The application of a good plaster is essential. The thumb and index finger must oppose. Use of the hand in plaster is essential; very little physiotherapy is required.

COMPLICATION

Non-union occurs in less than 10% of patients. Usually due to patient not reporting injury for several weeks. Early immobilization is essential.

COMMON FRACTURES—(TRAUMATIC)

Fractures of the hip and thigh	Usual age-group	How injury occurs	Most usual method of fixation	Movements begun	Complications	Results and Comments
UPPER FEMUR —Subcapital (intracapsular)	Elderly	Fall, quite often a minor one	1. Prosthesis or	Immediately; partial weight-bearing 1 week to full weight-bearing		Good if fixation holds and bony necrosis does not occur
			2. Internal fixation (Moore's pin)	Immediately; weight-bearing		
—Mid-cervical (intracapsular)	Elderly	Fall, quite often a minor one	1. Internal fixation (flanged pin) or	Immediately; full weight-bearing 12–16 weeks	Fixation or fracture moving causing non-union Avascular necrosis (early or delayed)	
			2. Internal fixation (Moore's pins)	Immediately; partial weight-bearing or full weight-bearing		
—Basal (intracapsular)	Elderly	Fall, quite often a minor one	Internal fixation (nail and plate)	Immediately; full weight-bearing 12–16 weeks	Failure of fixation	Good if fixation holds
—Per-trochanteric (extra capsular)	Elderly	Fall	1. Internal fixation (nail and plate) or	Immediately; non-weight-bearing to full weight-bearing 12–16 weeks		
			2. Traction 10–12 weeks	Immediately to lower leg etc.	Non-union or poor alignment	Seldom used now, loss of range and power in hip and knee
SHAFT	Young adult	Direct blow (e.g. road traffic accident)	1. Traction 3 months. Traction 2 months and special caliper for 1 month or	Immediately to foot; knee at 8–12 weeks; full weight-bearing 16–20 weeks	Non-union. Callus formation causing tethering of quadriceps	Good results (if union achieved) in the young

2.	Intramedullary nail or nails and plates or nails and plates or wires *or*	Immediately; non-weight-bearing 2–3 weeks; full weight-bearing 6–12 weeks		Elderly patients lose range in hip and knee
3.	Plating and wire bands usually with groin to toe plaster *or*	Dependent on external fixation; full weight-bearing at 12–16 weeks	Non-union	Good
4.	Compression plating	Immediately; non-weight-bearing 12–14 weeks and use of special caliper		

Notes

UPPER FEMUR FRACTURES

These patients are usually elderly. Prolonged bed-rest would often mean that the muscles atrophy and the joints stiffen. Generally their health would deteriorate. Therefore internal fixation is used. Early exercise and ambulation is encouraged.

RANGE

Usually these patients only want to be able to enjoy 'quiet' living, i.e. the ability to sit (90° of hip flexion), to stand and walk (some extension of hip if possible), toileting (30° abduction). A much greater range is desirable, but not essential.

POWER

Personal independence is only possible if the muscle power is sufficient to perform the action. Encouragement to keep practising sitting, standing or walking is very important. The quadriceps hamstring and glutei muscle groups are the most important ones to maintain.

COMPLICATIONS

Intracapsular fractures. Avascular necrosis. In the elderly the blood supply to the head of the femur is mainly from the capsular blood vessels. A fracture severs this supply. Internal fixation is designed to keep the bone fragments in close contact and in the hope that a blood supply can be established. However, the fragments often separate and

a slow necrosis occurs resulting in a collapse of the bony union one or two years later.

Extracapsular fractures. Failures of fixation. A very accurate bone alignment is required if the stresses on the fixator are not to be too great. This is not always possible and the metal may work loose or break.

FEMORAL SHAFT FRACTURES

These are usually the result of accidents or severe violence. There can be a clean break or a very comminuted fracture. The type of fracture will determine the method of fixation.

RANGE

Knee movements are often limited after these fractures. This may be due to the involvement of the quadriceps muscle in the fracture callus. A quadriceps-plasty may be required at some future time to overcome this. If this complication does not arise, knee range usually becomes normal.

POWER

The quadriceps muscle atrophies very quickly. It is important to encourage its use as quickly as possible after injury.

COMPLICATIONS

Non-union. This could be caused by over-traction, or a failure of the internal fixation to keep the bone ends in close contact.

COMMON FRACTURES—(TRAUMATIC)

Fractures of the region of the knee	Usual age-group	How injury occurs	Most usual method of fixation	Movements begun	Complications	Results and comments
SUPRA-CONDYLAR (Lower end of femur)	Any	Direct blow	1. Traction 3 months	Immediately static exercises all movements that are permitted; weight-bearing 3 months	Tibial nerve and popliteal artery	Gross loss of knee movements
			2. Compression plating or screwing	Immediately; weight-bearing 3 months		Some loss of knee movements
PATELLA	Any	Direct violence or stress	1. Plaster cylinder groin to ankle for 3 weeks *or*	Partial weight-bearing in plaster; knee movements at 3 weeks	Retropatellar arthritis Quadriceps lag	Young make full recovery, elderly lose some range and power
			2. Operation. Wiring or screwing and P.O.P. cylinder *or*			
			3. Operation. Excision of part or whole and plaster cylinder	Partial weight-bearing in plaster of Paris cylinder; knee movements at 4–6 weeks		Knee stiffness
TIBIAL-PLATEAU (Depression)	Adults	Fall	1. Plaster groin to ankle 8–12 weeks *or*	Knee movements as soon as plaster removed	Ruptured cruciate ligaments. Common peroneal nerve damage (in lateral plateau fracture)	If resulting depression is more than 1 cm, malfunction and instability follow. Knee stiffness
			2. Operation. Elevation of fragments and metal fixation P.O.P. groin to toe 6–8 weeks *or*	Immediately; non-weight-bearing to weight-bearing 6 weeks		
			3. None (elderly)			

Notes

FRACTURES OF THE FEMORAL CONDYLES OR TIBIAL PLATEAUX
Unless the bone architecture is restored after these fractures, the normal joint is deranged. Instability results in pain and loss of normal joint range. The type of trauma which gives rise to these injuries usually will have caused some degree of dislocation of the joint, often damaging the soft tissue very considerably.

RANGE
Full extension is the primary aim; without this the quadriceps muscles cannot act efficiently. A patient can learn 'to live with' a stiff straight knee, but a loss of 10°, or more, of extension creates a weak painful joint and a poor gait. It is seldom possible to regain full range movements after these fractures in the middle or older age-groups, so that full extension is the most important movement.

POWER
Controlled movements of the knee joint are essential in walking, sitting and standing. Whatever movements are restored to the joint, these are only as useful as the degree of muscle power controlling them. Every effort to maintain the power of the quadriceps muscle must be made, even if the knee joint cannot be moved because of fixation.

COMPLICATIONS
Cruciate ligament damage
These ligaments sustain some degree of stretching from injuries which result in tibial plateau fracture. They may even be ruptured.

Any ligament of the knee joint is liable to damage according to the way the injury is sustained.

Common peroneal nerve damage—This can occur at the time of an injury which causes a fracture to the lateral tibial plateau or a fractured neck of fibula.

FRACTURE OF PATELLA
The patella is a sesamoid bone in the tendon of the quadriceps femoris. It alters the angle of pull of the muscle. Whenever possible it is repaired. It requires a very firm internal fixation after a fracture. If it is severely comminuted it is partly or totally removed (it often re-forms). After reduction the posterior surface must be smooth or retropatellar arthritis develops.

It is important to keep the quadriceps muscles as strong as possible. A 'lag' occurs if the patella is removed because of the change in the angle pull of the muscle. This 'lag', or loss of full extension, is a feature of most fractures of the patella in the early stages of rehabilitation and must be overcome if the knee is to regain full stability.

COMMON FRACTURES—(TRAUMATIC)

Fractures of the Tibia and Fibula	Usual age-group	How injury occurs	Most usual method of fixation	Movements begun	Complications	Results and comments
SHAFT —TIBIA (undisplaced)	Any	Direct violence	1. Groin to toe plaster 8–12 weeks, below knee P.O.P for further 4 weeks *or* 2. Medullary nail	Knee movements as soon as plaster shortened Knee and ankle movements 7–10 days; non-weight-bearing to weight-bearing 10–12 weeks	Non-union	Good results in the younger age-groups
TIBIA AND FIBULA (SHAFTS) (*See Plate 11/5*)	Any	Direct or indirect violence	1. Groin to toe plaster 10–14 weeks *or* 2. Plating and groin to toe plaster 10–14 weeks *or*	Knee and ankle movements when plaster removed; weight-bearing in plaster 8–12 weeks; full weight-bearing 12–16 weeks	Non-union	Slow, usually good results in time
			3. Compression plating	Immediately; non-weight-bearing 12–14 weeks in special caliper	Non-union, common peroneal nerve compression	Good results. Loss of full dorsiflexion of ankle sometimes
—Lateral malleolus (with little or no displacement) (*See Plate 11/6*)	Any	Inversion injury	1. Strapping *or*	Immediately; weight-bearing		Excellent results
			2. Below knee plaster 4 weeks	Weight-bearing in plaster of paris; exercises when plaster removed		Excellent results
—Medial malleolus	Any	Eversion injury	1. Below knee plaster 4–6 weeks *or* 2. Operation. Screwing and below knee plaster 4–6 weeks	Walk in plaster at 2 weeks	Medial ligament damage leaving the joint unstable	Good if mortice is re-established
—Both malleoli (with disruption of the mortice) (*See Plate 11/7*)	Any	Jumping from a height onto the heels	1. Below knee plaster (always for children) *or* 2. Operation. Screwing and below knee plaster 8–10 weeks *or* 3. Operation. Compression screws	Walking in plaster 8–10 weeks Walking in plaster 6–8 weeks Immediate exercises, non-weight-bearing to weight-bearing 8–10 weeks		Children do well. Results depend on the degree of perfection of the joint reconstruction. The older the patient the greater the loss of joint movements. Balance impaired

				Immediate exercises; weight-bearing Walk in plaster of paris	If there is a loss of subtaloid movement, the patient should not work above ground level again
CALCANEUM	Adult	Jumping from a height onto the heels	1. Strapping or 2. Below knee plaster 8–12 weeks		
METATARSALS	Adult	Stress or weight falling on foot	Below knee plaster 4–6 weeks	Weight-bearing in plaster	Excellent results
—5th	Adult	Inversion injury	Strapping 1 week	Normal use	

Notes

FRACTURES OF THE SHAFT OF THE TIBIA AND FIBULA
There are many different types of fracture that can occur, from a simple transverse fracture of the tibia without displacement, to a severely comminuted fracture of both bones.

COMPLICATION
Non-union. This is quite common, especially in young men. A secondary operative procedure, such as a bone graft or internal fixation, may have to be performed. Whilst compression plating has reduced the percentage of non-union results, it has its own complication of a 'dropped foot'. It is difficult to say whether this is a result of pressure on the common peroneal nerve by the special walking caliper, or as a result of the operative technique. Full recovery of the nerve lesion may take several months.

FRACTURES OF THE ANKLE AND HINDFOOT
The function of the foot on the lower leg is to perform the actions required for propulsion of the body over uneven surfaces and at varying speeds. The injuries that can be sustained vary from a simple strain to complex fracture-dislocations involving one or more joints. Unless the bone and joint architecture can be restored to normal, the function of the foot is restricted and usually painful.

RANGE
Inversion and eversion are the most important movements to restore. Without them walking on uneven surfaces is painful or even impossible.

Plantarflexion is required to give the 'push off' range for the action of the calf and flexor hallucis longus muscles, which together make the normal gait. The loss of dorsiflexion can be accommodated by raising the heel of the shoe.

POWER
Controlled movement is more important than range. The whole body-weight rests on the forefoot during walking and running, and unless the ankle and hindfoot are controlled there is a great incapacity.

COMPLICATIONS
There are no specific immediate complications. However, these injuries are often disabling and result in patients being unable to resume their normal work again, e.g. calcaneal fractures which involve the subtaloid joint may necessitate a scaffolder giving up climbing.

Arthritis often develops where articular surfaces have been damaged. Ligaments may be partially or totally ruptured, giving rise to painful instability. Loss of normal joint architecture may make for either limited or unstable movements, which are often painful.

FRACTURES OF THE METATARSALS
These are minor injuries and repair well with no disability. Most can be treated by strapping and immediate use.

COMMON FRACTURES—(TRAUMATIC)

Fractures of the pelvis	Usual age-group	How injury occurs	Most usual method of fixation	Movements begun	Complications	Results and comments
1. Single —Wing of ilium. Rami of either pubis or ilium	Adult	Crush injury or direct blow	Bed-rest for 2–7 days	Bed exercises; weight-bearing 2–7 days		Good. Pain can persist for several weeks
2. Multiple —Two rami on same side with displacement	Adult	Crush injury, Bed-rest with skin traction on leg of affected side (2–3 weeks) falling from a height on to one foot		When traction removed gentle non-weight-bearing exercises; avoid straight leg raising in early stages; partial weight-bearing 3–4 weeks		
Four rami (butterfly fracture)	Adult	Crush injury	Operation. To stabilize fragments (wire or plates) and a pelvic sling	None until united; then gentle non-weight-bearing exercises; straight leg raising delayed for 6–8 weeks; walking at 8–12 weeks	Urethra or bladder damage	Slow but good
ACETABULUM —Posterior rim (and posterior dislocation of hip)	Adult	Blow on knee when leg is flexed and adducted	1. Reduction of dislocation. Traction for 4–6 weeks or 2. Large fragments screwed and traction for 4–6 weeks	Gentle non-weight-bearing exercises when traction is removed; weight-bearing 5–7 weeks	Sciatic nerve palsy, usually recovers quickly	Excellent in the young. Good in the elderly

—	—	—	—	—	—	—
—Comminuted (and central dislocation of hip)	Adult	Blow or fall on great trochanter	Reduction of dislocation by traction from a pin in the greater trochanter 6–8 weeks (Reduction is not possible because of rotation of fragments.) Traction for 6–10 weeks	Gentle non-weight-bearing exercises when traction is removed; partial weight-bearing 7–11 weeks; full weight-bearing 9–13 weeks	Osteoarthrosis inevitable. Possible damage to pelvic contents	Much better than one expects. The young make a very good recovery but often have osteo-arthrosis later in life. If pain persists further surgery may be required.
—Iliopubic (and central dislocation of hip)					Osteoarthrosis occasionally. Possible damage to pelvic contents	

stages movements of the hip are not possible, because of the traction needed to retain the reduction of the dislocation and the time necessary for the capsular ligamentous damage to repair. When hip movement is permitted, care should be taken to avoid reproducing the action which preceded the dislocation as this may cause further soft tissue damage and even a re-dislocation of the joint. (E.g. a posterior dislocation occurs when the hip is flexed and adducted, and therefore these movements should only be performed with care.)

The speed at which exercise therapy is progressed is best left to the patient. Any pain he experiences should be considered an indication that the progression has been too fast. Young people recover well. Patients within the older age-group are usually left with some loss of movement in the hip.

COMPLICATIONS
Osteoarthrosis is an inevitable long-term result. However, it is only an immediate problem with the elderly, many of whom already had some osteoarthritic changes present in the joint. Sciatic nerve palsy can occur with posterior dislocations, but this usually recovers quickly and spontaneously. Damage to internal organs may have occurred as a result of the compression force that was exerted at the time of the injury.

Notes

PELVIC GIRDLE
A single fracture of the pelvic girdle (i.e. one ramus, or the winging of the ilium) does not significantly alter the stability of the pelvis. Early ambulation and exercise should be encouraged.

Multiple fractures (i.e. two rami on the same side, or all four rami) render the pelvic girdle unstable. Therefore weight-bearing must be delayed until there is bony union. The strong pull of the muscles attached to these bones makes displacement severe. Union is essential before exercises are given. It must be remembered that straight-leg raising, especially if performed in the supine posture, is an advanced type of exercise for these patients in view of the length of the lever. This type of exercise should be delayed until the bony union is sufficiently firm to withstand the strain.

COMPLICATIONS
There is always a danger that the internal organs may have been damaged at the time of the accident. The urethra and bladder are particularly vulnerable. The final diameters of the pelvis are particularly important to females of child-bearing age.

ACETABULUM
These fractures occur with dislocations of the hip joint. In the early

COMMON FRACTURES—(TRAUMATIC)

Fractures of the Spine	Usual age-group	How injury occurs	Most usual method of fixation	Movements begun	Complications	Results and comments
VERTEBRAL BODIES —Severe lesions with neurological involvement (see Chapters VIII–X, *Neurology for Physiotherapists*)						
—anterior wedging (minor)	Adult	Flexion injury	1. Bed-rest for few days *or* 2. Plaster corset	Graduated extension exercises		Good result if only one vertebra is affected. Occasionally a fusion operation is needed if pain persists
VERTEBRAL ARCH —transverse process —spinous process	Adult	Avulsion fracture due to violent muscle action	Continued activity	Encourage movement		Good. Full recovery

Notes

FRACTURES OF THE VERTEBRAE

Vertebral bodies. Minor crush injuries to vertebral bodies are usually best treated by early ambulation and exercise. It is important to reassure the patient that his injury is only a minor one, as the phrase 'broken back' or 'fractured spine' conjures up a very serious implication to most patients.

COMPLICATIONS

Persistent pain can be a feature and sometimes a fusion of two or three vertebrae may be necessary to overcome this. The greatest complication is the patient's fear that he may be permanently disabled.

VERTEBRAL ARCH

These fractures are often very painful since they are frequently aggravated with soft tissue damage. The best treatment for them is analgesics and normal activity. Bed-rest tends to prolong the painful period. Local treatment may be given as for any contusion.

COMPLICATIONS

None, so long as the patient's natural apprehension can be overcome and free active movement re-established.

Soft tissue injuries (Chapters 7 and 8)

BIBLIOGRAPHY

Armstrong, J. R. *Lumbar Disc Lesions*. Churchill Livingstone, 3rd ed. 1965.

Brain (Lord). *Clinical Neurology* (revised by R. Bannister). Oxford Medical Publications, 4th ed. 1973.

Cailliet, R. *Low Back Pain Syndrome*. Blackwell Scientific Publications, 2nd ed. 1968.

Cailliet, R. *Neck and Arm Pain*. Blackwell Scientific Publications, 1964.

Cailliet, R. *Shoulder Pain*. Blackwell Scientific Publications, 1966.

Cyriax, J. *The Slipped Disc*. Gower Press, 1970.

Featherstone, D. *Sports Injuries: their prevention and treatment*. John Wright, 1957.

Gray's Anatomy: illustrated and applied (edited by R. Warwick). Longman, 35th ed. 1973.

London, P. S. *Practical Guide to the Care of the Injured*. Churchill Livingstone, 1967.

MacConaill, M. A. and Basmajian, R. S. *Muscles and Movements*. Williams & Watkins, 1969.

Robbins, S. L. and Angell, L. M. *Basic Pathology*. W. B. Saunders, 1971.

Shands, A. R. *Handbook of Orthopaedic Surgery* (edited by R. B. Raney and H. R. Brashear). C. V. Mosley, 8th ed. 1972.

Smillie, I. S. *Injuries of the Knee Joint*. Churchill Livingstone, 4th ed. 1970.

Williams, J. G. P. (ed.). *Sports Medicine*. Edward Arnold, 1962.

Major multiple injuries (Chapter 9)

REFERENCES

d'Abreu, A. L. and Clarke, D. B. 'Thoracic Injuries' in *Modern Trends in Accident Surgery and Medicine*, Vol. 2 (edited by P. S. London). Butterworth, 1972.

Proctor, H. and Lockhart, P. 'Head Injuries: problems of the crippled survivors', *ibid*.

Porter, N. F. 'Advances in the Care of the Injured'. *The Practitioner*, No. 1252 Vol. 209, p. 544, 1972.

BIBLIOGRAPHY

Cash, J. E. (ed.). *Neurology for Physiotherapists*. 'Head Injuries' by E. L. Renfrew. Faber & Faber, 1974.

Bibliographies and References

Cash, J. E. (ed.). *Chest, Heart and Vascular Disorders for Physiotherapists.* 'Intensive Care' by P. J. Waddington. Faber & Faber, 1975.
Cash, J. E. *A Textbook of Medical Conditions for Physiotherapists.* 'Burns' by R. Wootton. Faber & Faber, 5th ed. 1976.

The physiotherapist's approach
to athletic and sports injuries (Chapter 9)

REFERENCE

Williams, J. G. P. (ed.). *Sports Medicine.* Edward Arnold, 1962.

BIBLIOGRAPHY

Dyson, G. H. G. *The Mechanics of Athletics.* University of London Press, 6th ed. 1973.
Featherstone, D. F. *Sports Injuries: their prevention and treatment.* John Wright, 1957.
Morgan, R. E. and Adamson, G. T. *Circuit Training.* G. Ball & Sons, 2nd ed. 1961.

Fractures (Chapter 10)

BIBLIOGRAPHY

Adams, J. Crawford. *Outline of Orthopaedics.* Churchill Livingstone, 7th ed. 1971.
Bloom, W. and Fawcett, D. W. *A Textbook of Histology.* W. B. Saunders, 9th ed. 1968.
Charnley, J. *The Closed Treatment of Common Fractures.* Churchill Livingstone, 3rd ed. 1961.
Cruikshank, B. *et al. Human Histology.* Churchill Livingstone, 2nd ed. 1968.
Guyton, A. C. *Textbook of Medical Physiology.* W. B. Saunders, 4th ed. 1971.
London, P. S. *Practical Guide to the Care of the Injured.* Churchill Livingstone, 1967.
Mercer, Sir Walter and Duthie, R. B. *Orthopaedic Surgery.* Edward Arnold, 6th ed. 1964.
Muller, M. E., Allgöwer, M. and Willenegger, H. *Manual of Internal Fixation.* Springer Verlag, Berlin, 1970.
de Palma, A. F. *The Management of Fractures and Dislocations,* Vol. I and II. W. B. Saunders, 2nd ed. 1970.
Passmore, R. and Robson, J. S. *A Companion to Medical Studies,* Vol. I. Blackwell Scientific Publications, 1968.

Bibliographies and References

Wiles, P. and Sweetnam, R. *Essentials of Orthopaedics*. Churchill Livingstone, 4th ed. 1965.

Wiles, P. and Sweetnam, R. *Fractures, Dislocations and Sprains*. Churchill Livingstone, 2nd ed. 1969.

Williams, J. G. P. (ed.). *Sports Medicine*. Edward Arnold, 1962.

CHAPTER 12

Amputations

BRIDGET DAVIS, MCSP, HT, ONC

Amputation of a limb performed for vascular disorders when other treatment has proved ineffective, or amputation as a result of trauma, malignancy or deformity should be accepted as a positive form of treatment, relieving the patient of a painful, useless, dangerous and often infected extremity.

After amputation has been performed, the patient can be rehabilitated to a fully independent life, return to work, and in time become as active as he was prior to amputation, depending upon his general condition.

The amputee needs time and help to overcome the psychological shock resulting from the loss of a limb. He realizes that he is different from other people and, more important, that this difference will be apparent. He will be uncertain of his future and will need encouragement from all members of the rehabilitation team: the surgeon, nursing staff, physiotherapists, occupational therapists, social workers, the medical officer at the Limb Fitting Centre, prosthetist and the patient's general practitioner. All these people must work in close co-operation with one another.

Rehabilitation is one continual process from the time the surgeon decides to amputate, until such time that the patient is independent with his definitive prosthesis. This may take six months, although the patient is unlikely to remain in hospital for the whole of this period.

Amputations of upper and lower limbs involve differences in cause, age-group and rehabilitation, and so will be considered separately. The ratio of lower limb to upper limb amputees is of the order of 9 to 1.

LOWER LIMB AMPUTATIONS

This is the larger group of amputees and these patients are seen in greater numbers by physiotherapists.

Indications for amputation

The causes of lower limb amputation together with the approximate percentage of cases are as follows:

Peripheral vascular disease and diabetes 73
Trauma 12
Malignancy 6
Congenital deformities 2
Other 7

It is seen that peripheral vascular disease and diabetic gangrene (diseases associated with the elderly), account for the majority of lower limb amputations, and accordingly in any one year 70% of new lower limb amputees are over the age of 60. These patients often have many of the other problems associated with the elderly: cardiac involvement, low exercise tolerance, arteriosclerosis of the cerebral vessels causing possible hemiplegia and diminished mental ability, poor respiratory function, reduced visual acuity, poor healing, osteoarthrosis and neuropathy.

Traumatic amputations more commonly affect the younger age-groups and are mostly necessitated by road traffic accidents and industrial injuries.

Malignant disease is a reason for amputation also in the patients in the younger age-groups.

Amputations for congenital deformity and limb length discrepancies are usually performed on children and young adults. This is best delayed until the patient is old enough to decide for himself that he wishes to have the operation performed.

The limb fitting service

Before discussing the treatment of the amputee, it is important that the student should understand something of the prosthetic service available to the patient. This obviously varies in different countries, but in the United Kingdom a uniform and comprehensive service is offered to all amputees.

Amputations

There are 26 Limb Fitting Centres throughout England, Wales and Northern Ireland which are administered directly by the Department of Health and Social Security. There are also five centres in Scotland for which the Scottish Home and Health Department is responsible. The patient is referred to his nearest centre by the surgeon at the hospital at which he had his amputation. There he is seen by a Medical Officer who will be responsible for his limb fitting programme and prosthetic rehabilitation. The patient is examined, assessed and usually measured for his temporary prosthesis on his first visit.

The patient remains under the care of the Artificial Limb Fitting Service all his life, for he will continually require repairs and replacement of his artificial limb. He will also be supplied with sufficient woollen or cotton stump socks, bandages, walking aids and other appliances as he requires them.

Should the patient move to another part of the country he is transferred to his nearest Regional Limb Fitting Centre.

All artificial limbs are made by independent manufacturers under contract to the Department of Health and Social Security.

Surgery and levels of amputation

Whatever the pathology predisposing to amputation, there are many factors which will influence the surgeon in his selection of level of amputation. As well as the pathology, the surgeon will also consider factors such as surgical techniques, viability of tissue, prostheses and not least important the patient's particular needs, taking into account his occupation, importance of good cosmesis, age and sex.

HINDQUARTER AMPUTATION
This amputation is performed almost solely for malignancy as a life-saving procedure and here, obviously, the pathological factors are of prime importance. The surgeon has no choice but to remove the entire limb and part of the ilium, pubis, ischium and sacrum on that side, leaving peritoneum, muscle and fascia to cover and support the internal organs.

HIP DISARTICULATION
This procedure is commonly performed in cases of malignancy; it may also be necessary following excessive trauma but is seldom done for

vascular insufficiency. The limb is disarticulated at the hip-joint and the bony pelvis is left intact, thus producing a good weight-bearing platform.

MID-THIGH AMPUTATION

This is the amputation which is perhaps most commonly seen in the elderly group of patients. In the patient with vascular disease, an above-knee amputation is one in which primary healing occurs more readily than the through-knee or below-knee amputation. However, compared with these other levels, the above-knee amputee will have more difficulty in learning to control his prosthesis and in achieving a good gait and, in the case of the elderly patient, the attainment of total independence will be more of a problem. Proprioception from the knee-joint will be lost and the patient must bear weight on the prosthesis at the ischial tuberosity. Hip flexion contractures occur very easily unless care is taken to prevent them, the shorter stumps tending to become flexed and abducted (due particularly to the strong pull of tensor fascia lata). The longer above-knee stumps by contrast tend to become flexed and adducted (there will be more of the adductor group intact and these muscles have a mechanical advantage over the pull of the short tensor fascia lata).

The surgeon makes the above-knee stump as long as possible, but must leave $4\frac{1}{2}$–5 inches (115–130 mm) between the end of the stump and the knee axis in order to leave space for the knee control mechanisms to be put into the prosthesis. If, however, there is a hip flexion contracture, a long stump is a disadvantage as the end of the long stump magnifies the contracture and the prosthesis will be very bulky to accommodate this.

Many surgeons use the myoplastic technique or a myodesis in which muscle groups are sutured together over the bone end or attached to the bone at physiological tension. The muscles therefore retain their contractile property, circulation to the stump is improved, and the stump will be more powerful in the control of a prosthesis.

AMPUTATION AT KNEE-JOINT LEVEL

This includes disarticulation of the knee and the Gritti-Stokes amputation. In the former, the tibia together with the fibula is disarticulated at the knee-joint. The patella is retained and the patellar tendon is sutured to the anterior cruciate ligament, the hamstrings are sutured to the posterior cruciate ligament and so act as hip extensors. A strong powerful stump results with no muscle imbalance, and full end bearing is possible on the broad expanse of the femoral condyles. Most of the proprioception of the knee-joint is retained.

In the Gritti-Stokes technique, the femur is sectioned transversely through the condyles, the articular surface of the patella is shaved off and the patella positioned at the distal end of the femur. Bony union should occur, and weight is taken on the patella.

Full end bearing is possible on the knee disarticulation, but due to the relatively smaller weight-bearing surface in the Gritti-Stokes amputation, this is often not possible and a certain amount of weight must be taken through the ischial tuberosity. However, the Gritti-Stokes amputation necessitates smaller skin flaps with better vascular nutrition and therefore primary healing is more certain.

BELOW-KNEE AMPUTATION

If at all possible, the surgeon will elect to perform a below-knee amputation. The great advantage is that the normal knee-joint with its proprioception is retained and therefore balance and a good gait pattern will be more easily attained. The optimum level is $5\frac{1}{2}$ inches (140 mm) below the tibial plateau, although a patient with a slightly shorter stump would still achieve good function with a prosthesis.

The fibula is sectioned slightly more proximally than the tibia, and the end of the tibia is bevelled to avoid a prominent bone end. Frequently a myoplastic technique is used, resulting in the advantages previously described.

SYMES AMPUTATION

This involves disarticulation at the ankle-joint and removal of the medial and lateral malleoli to the level of the articular surface of the tibia. This amputation is not done in vascular conditions, as a higher level will always be necessary due to insufficient blood supply. Good end bearing is possible, the heel pad being sutured into position over the distal end of the tibia and fibula.

FOOT AMPUTATIONS

Trans- and midtarsal amputations result in relatively little locomotor difficulty, the main problem being that of the provision of satisfactory footwear.

PHYSIOTHERAPY

The physiotherapist's role in the rehabilitation of the amputee can be considered in three stages: pre-operative, postoperative (pre-prosthetic), and prosthetic.

Again it must be emphasized that rehabilitation is one continual process, the final goal for the patient being independence on his definitive prosthesis and a return to normal activities, within the limitations of his age and condition.

Pre-operative stage

Treatment at this stage is of course most applicable to the patient with vascular disease, and in these cases a pre-operative exercise programme is very valuable. Many of these patients have been at home or in hospital confined to bed or to a chair because of a lesion of the foot, gangrene or ischaemic pain. If the patient has been walking at all he will only have been hobbling from one room to another, the joints of the affected leg will be held in a position of flexion (the reflex response to pain) and his general condition will be poor.

The physiotherapist should assess the patient's physical abilities and also take into account his mental attitude and home conditions. On the basis of this assessment she will commence and progress the physical treatment programme, at all times with reference to the surgeon, nursing staff and other members of the rehabilitation team.

During the pre-operative stage, the patient has the opportunity to adapt to his changing circumstances, to learn to know the staff who are concerned in his rehabilitation, and perhaps to meet other amputees who are progressing towards independence. The psychological aspect is very important and the physiotherapist can do much to help and motivate the patient.

Depending upon the time available and the general condition of the patient, the following should be included in the treatment programme:

(*i*) Strengthening exercises for the upper trunk and upper limbs to facilitate crutch walking, transfers and for moving up and down the bed.

(*ii*) Strengthening and mobilizing exercises for the lower trunk, necessary for all activities, rolling, sitting up, walking.

(*iii*) Strengthening exercises for the unaffected leg for crutch walking, standing, transferring.

(*iv*) Exercises for the affected leg to increase the range of movement and improve stability of those joints which will remain after amputation.

(*v*) Crutch walking, if possible, non weight-bearing with the affected leg.

(*vi*) Maximal independence including ability to move about the bed using the unaffected leg, rolling, prone lying.

(*vii*) It is important to teach wheelchair activities even though it is hoped that the patient will ultimately achieve independence on a prosthesis. A few weeks will elapse before he receives this and in the meantime he should be encouraged to be as independent as possible. Many of the elderly patients do not manage with any degree of safety on crutches.

Postoperative stage

The aims of treatment at this stage are:
   (*i*) prevention of joint contractures;
   (*ii*) to strengthen and co-ordinate the muscles controlling the stump;
   (*iii*) to strengthen and mobilize the unaffected leg;
   (*iv*) to strengthen and mobilize the trunk;
   (*v*) to teach the patient to regain independence in functional activities;
   (*vi*) to control oedema of the stump.

Physiotherapy will be commenced the day following operation. It should always be remembered that most of the patients undergoing amputation for vascular reasons have been heavy smokers for many years, therefore chest complications are not uncommon. Routine postoperative breathing exercises should be commenced on the first day.

PREVENTION OF CONTRACTURES

Attention should be given to the position of the patient in bed. The stump should lie parallel to the unaffected leg with the joints extended. There should be no pillow under the stump and there should be fracture boards beneath the mattress. Both physiotherapists and nursing staff should keep a check on the patient's position. The patient should understand its importance and be encouraged to maintain it.

A routine of prone lying, with all joints in as much extension as possible, is commenced as soon as the patient can tolerate it, usually on the third postoperative day, ideally for 15 to 20 minutes, three times daily. If the patient is unable to lie prone because of cardiac or respiratory problems, he should lie supine for as long as he can tolerate it, again two or three times a day.

STRENGTHENING OF THE STUMP

Isometric work for the muscles of the stump is started three days after operation. As the wound heals, manually resisted isotonic work can be given and gradually progressed. It is inadvisable, particularly when the myoplastic technique has been used, to give strong resisted work until about 14 days after surgery, as there will be much suture material in the wound and care must be taken not to pull on this.

The physiotherapist must at all times watch for any muscle imbalance and pay particular attention to the weaker groups, which will most likely be the extensors of the hip and knee and possibly the hip adductors, in fact, those muscles necessary to oppose a potential contracture (p. 297). Stability of all joints of the stump will be essential in the effective control of a prosthesis.

STRENGTHENING AND MOBILIZING THE UNAFFECTED LEG

Strong isometric 'holds' with the hip and knee in extension (see Plate 12/1) are useful in helping to retain the supportive function of the leg, and this isometric work together with resisted isotonic exercises can be started the day following operation. During the next few days, as the patient's general condition improves, these exercises are progressed. When the sutures are removed from the stump and firm bandaging has been commenced, standing and walking in the parallel bars and on crutches is encouraged, emphasis being placed on hip extension.

TO STRENGTHEN AND MOBILIZE THE TRUNK

Rolling (see Plates 12/4, 12/5) and 'bridging' (see Plate 12/2) exercises can be commenced on the first day, and on about the third day when the patient is able to sit on the edge of his bed, resisted sitting balance work is given (see Plates 12/6, 12/7). As soon as the patient is able to go to the physiotherapy department, the resisted trunk exercises are progressed on mats together with reciprocal leg activity, and sitting balance improved. Attention is also given to the upper trunk and upper limbs (weight and pulley systems are useful for this, see Plates 12/3, 12/8). Group work can be of value although elderly patients benefit more from individual treatment sessions, and two of these sessions daily in the physiotherapy department with perhaps occupational therapy as well is usually an adequate programme for these patients.

INDEPENDENCE IN FUNCTIONAL ACTIVITIES
At all times the patient must be encouraged to be as independent as possible. His treatment programme should progress in the physiotherapy department as soon as he is fit enough to leave the ward, usually about the fourth day. He should dress himself in the morning (sometimes it is necessary for the occupational therapist to give dressing practice) and he should wear a good walking shoe on the unaffected leg. Basic wheelchair independence is taught including transfers from bed to chair and from chair to lavatory, and he should be able to wheel himself around the ward and if possible to the physiotherapy department.

CONTROL OF OEDEMA
When the sutures have been removed (between 14 and 21 days after amputation) firm stump bandaging must be commenced. The purpose of this is to disperse the terminal oedema which is always present, particularly in the above- and below-knee stumps.

It is essential that the oedema is reduced as quickly as possible so that the stump assumes its ultimate size quickly and the limb fitting programme is not delayed. Firm bandaging conditions the stump to constant all-round pressure which the patient will experience when wearing a prosthesis.

Above-knee or through-knee stumps require 5 yards (4·5 metres) of 6 inch (15 cm) wide 'Elset' or crepe bandage.

It is important that most pressure is applied at the distal end of the stump, and least pressure proximally. No constricting turns should be made, all should be kept diagonal, and the bandage must go well up into the groin (see Figs. 12/1-12/5).

The bandage is commenced anteriorly on the stump in the inguinal region, the patient fixing the end with his thumbs. It then passes over the end of the stump and up to the gluteal fold posteriorly, the patient fixing this turn with his fingers (Fig. 12/1). The bandage is returned anteriorly over the end of the stump on the lateral side and again posteriorly over the end medially (see Fig. 12/2). The bandage is now brought round the lateral aspect of the stump and carried downwards anteriorly to the medial side of the distal end (Fig. 12/3). A turn is taken around the end of the stump posteriorly and then diagonally up proximally to the medial side anteriorly (Fig. 12/3). This figure-of-eight is repeated, gradually working up the stump. In order to help

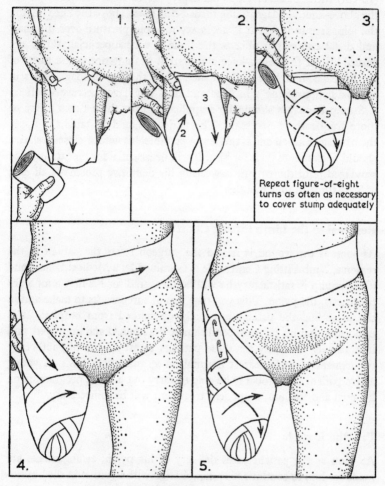

Figs. 12/1–5 Bandaging an above-knee stump.

secure the bandage, one or two turns are taken around the waist, posteriorly over the buttock, forwards around the waist and down to the stump posterolaterally, preventing the stump being pulled into flexion (Fig. 12/4). When bandaging the long through-knee stump it is not usually necessary to take the turns around the waist.

Below-knee and Symes stumps require 5 yards (4·5 metres) of 4 inch (10 cm) wide 'Elset' or crepe bandage. The turns are the same as for the above-knee bandage, fixing turns being taken above the knee leaving the joint free to move. It is necessary to avoid pressure over the shaft and distal end of the tibia as the bone is very superficial. When the suture line of the below-knee amputation lies anteriorly, the turns of the bandage should be made in such a way that the bandage assists in approximation of the skin flaps and does not have the reverse effect.

Stump bandages should be reapplied at least three times a day or more frequently if necessary. The patient should be taught to apply the bandage himself and if this is not possible, his wife or closest relative should be taught to do it for him. It will be essential for the stump to be bandaged until the patient is wearing his definitive prosthesis all day, at least three to four months.

Referral to the Limb Fitting Centre

As soon as the wound is healed the surgeon refers the patient to the regional Limb Fitting Centre. He is examined by a Medical Officer and if the stump is satisfactory he will be measured for his first temporary prosthesis, the pylon. This will take two or three weeks to make and in the meantime the patient is usually discharged from hospital. It is important that his physical condition be maintained and improved, and it is usually necessary for these patients to attend the physiotherapy department of their nearest hospital on an outpatient basis. A young active patient will probably be able to carry out a home programme on his own and for him, outpatient treatment will be unnecessary.

Prosthetic stage

As soon as the patient takes delivery of his pylon, arrangements are made for him to continue his rehabilitation with it, either in the physio-therapy department of his original hospital or in the department at the Limb Fitting Centre. The patient must learn not only to walk safely and well but be able to put the pylon on independently, to stand up from a chair, climb stairs, walk up and down a slope, on rough ground and possibly manage public transport.

It is advisable for the patient to attend daily if possible for a whole or half-day session. Elderly patients frequently experience difficulty in tolerating the prosthesis, and unless they wear this regularly for the greater part of the day their performance on an artificial limb is certain to remain limited. During all stages of treatment, it should be remembered that many of these patients have undergone amputation for vascular conditions and therefore the other leg is likely also to be involved. It is important to observe the other leg and to make sure that any lesions of the foot are dressed and sufficiently protected by adequate footwear when commencing gait re-education (see chapters on Peripheral Vascular Disease in *Chest, Heart and Vascular Disorders for Physiotherapists*).

In teaching the patient a good gait pattern on his pylon, it is necessary to bear in mind the fact that the patient will of necessity have to walk with a stiff knee. Accordingly hip up-drawing on the side of the pylon must be stressed and the patient taught to bring the pylon forward without circumduction. All pylons have a type of knee mechanism which will only take the patient's weight if locked in extension. The knee lock can be released on sitting down. When the patient sits in a chair he puts his weight on the sound leg, releases the knee lock and sits down. On standing, he pushes on the arms of the chair, and with his weight on the sound leg and with the rocker base of the pylon on the ground, he extends his stump as he stands, so locking the joint. Alternatively, the patient can be taught to lock the pylon before standing and to release the lock only after he has sat down. On climbing stairs, the patient puts the sound leg up first and brings the pylon onto the same step. To descend, the pylon is lowered first, the sound leg following.

The pylon is suspended on the patient by a pelvic band and shoulder strap. There is a rocker base instead of a foot, which facilitates weight transference and good even gait (see Plate 12/9).

Although no allowances are made for cosmesis, the pylon is usually acceptable to the patient because it is functional and takes only two weeks to manufacture. It is lighter than a definitive prosthesis and because of the rocker base it is relatively easy for the patient to walk well. Usually two walking sticks are the only aids required.

After one or two weeks the patient is normally discharged from outpatient treatment and he continues using his pylon at home, wearing it daily, for the whole day. Some patients at this stage are able to return to work.

The patient is reviewed by the Medical Officer in four to six weeks' time, and if the stump has sufficiently reduced in size (bandaging is still being continued at night), a cast and measurements are taken for the definitive prosthesis. At present, this will take approximately three months to manufacture, with at least one fitting. On completion of the prosthesis, the patient is called up to the Limb Fitting Centre and if all is satisfactory, he takes delivery of the limb. He then reattends at an outpatient department as he did with his pylon, for final rehabilitation.

Again it will be necessary to teach the patient how to put on his new artificial limb and carry out all functional activities. His gait may be altered, for if he is an above- or through-knee amputee he may have been given a free-knee mechanism and he must learn to control the prosthesis accordingly. In this case, during the swing phase the prosthesis is brought forwards by hip flexion to heel strike, the stump is then extended strongly against the posterior wall of the socket of the prosthesis which will ensure that the limb is fully extended and so stable enough to take the patient's weight for the stance phase.

Stairs are negotiated in the same manner as with the pylon. A below-knee amputee will have to accustom himself to controlling his prosthesis with his normal knee-joint and musculature which probably will have become weak during the time spent on the pylon. Frequently the elderly amputee will be given a knee lock on his prosthesis, resulting in more stability.

It is advisable both with the pylon and the definitive limb to start the patient in the parallel bars, teaching the basic fundamentals of gait with good weight transference, and then to progress to walking with two sticks. Occasionally two tetrapods will be necessary. The patient should be encouraged not to look down at his feet when walking, although this is inevitable in the early stages as it will compensate for the total loss of proprioception in the joints of the amputated part of the limb. He must learn as soon as possible to feel with the remaining joints the positioning of the prosthesis in the gait sequence.

A patient should never be allowed to walk with crutches whilst wearing his prosthesis as he will tend to bear weight on the crutches and not on the artificial limb. Very occasionally it may be necessary to teach the patient to walk with a frame, although this should only be done when he has proved unsuccessful with other walking aids. It is not possible to attain a good gait when using a frame and the patient will always be dependent on this rather bulky aid.

Elderly patients, particularly those living on their own, should be taught how to get up from the floor should they have a fall. This is best done by showing the patient how to pull himself across the floor to some stable piece of furniture, e.g. sofa, armchair, bed, and then to get himself from the floor onto this. Double amputees are best advised to remove their prostheses first.

THE BILATERAL AMPUTEE

Occasionally as a result of trauma it will be necessary to amputate both lower limbs immediately. Unilateral amputees with vascular disease should be regarded as potential bilateral amputees within three years, depending upon the severity of the condition. It can be seen therefore, that it is not uncommon for the physiotherapist to be called upon to rehabilitate these severely disabled patients.

The pre- and postoperative treatment of the bilateral amputee follows that of the single amputee, although obviously he will be unable to walk on crutches or in the parallel bars. Particular attention must be paid to strengthening and mobilizing the upper limbs and trunk, and care taken to prevent flexion contractures of the hips developing whilst the patient waits for his pylons. These patients will all require a wheelchair and a suitable model must be ordered for the patient whilst he is in hospital. All wheelchair activities must be taught, including transfers, possibly with the use of a sliding board.

The temporary pylons that the patient receives, rocker pylons, are very much shorter than the patient's normal legs, being 18 to 24 inches (46 to 61 cm) high for the above-knee amputee and proportionately shorter for the through- and below-knee amputee. These short pylons lower the patient's centre of gravity and make balance easier. The patient takes weight on both ischial tuberosities and so in effect is walking upon two stilts. He does not have a normal foot on the ground feeding in sensory information and helping with balance. It will be appreciated that these patients require a longer period of prosthetic rehabilitation, frequently four to five weeks of daily attendance. (See Plates 12/10, 12/11, 12/12, 12/13.)

When the patient is mobile and competent on his pylons, he is reviewed by the Medical Officer who will decide whether the patient will be able to manage definitive prostheses, or whether he should remain in his wheelchair, walking on his pylons only in the house. If he receives definitive prostheses, these will tend to be shorter than his normal legs, but nonetheless, cosmetically acceptable. A further period of rehabilitation will be necessary on these.

Very occasionally a patient will not be fitted with prostheses, either as a single or as a bilateral amputee. He may have multiple disabilities including hemiplegia, blindness or rheumatoid arthritis, his social conditions may make it unrealistic for him to be mobile on prostheses, or he may himself elect not to be fitted. These patients will need to be rehabilitated to a wheelchair existence and adaptations in the home will have to be made where necessary.

Immediate postoperative fitting of prosthesis

In some hospitals and centres a slightly different postoperative routine is employed. While the patient is still under anaesthetic, the surgeon applies a rigid plaster of Paris socket to the stump over the dressing. To the end of this is incorporated a metal fitment to which can be attached a length of tubing and a prosthetic foot. The advantages of a plaster of Paris 'wrap' are firm control of the stump oedema with early maturation or shrinkage of the stump. The patient stands two to three days after surgery, but takes only minimal weight on the prosthesis. Other strengthening and mobilizing exercises are given as previously described.

After 14 days the plaster is removed and the sutures taken out, another plaster together with the prosthetic appliance is applied and rehabilitation continued. The patient progresses to walking on the prosthesis with elbow crutches, still only taking minimal weight on that side. At no time does the patient take full weight on this prosthesis, and he continues to walk with elbow crutches. After a further 14 days the plaster is removed and if the stump is satisfactory a cast is taken for a prosthesis.

With this method, earlier fitting of a definitive prosthesis is normally possible and the patient is rehabilitated in a shorter period of time. However, a closely co-ordinated team of specialists in the rehabilitation of amputees is necessary, and in order to reduce the risk of infection, patients need to be cared for in specialized units. It has been found that general surgical wards are not suitable for this regime.

UPPER LIMB AMPUTATIONS

Patients who undergo amputation of the upper limb, do so most commonly as a result of trauma from accidents at work or road accidents, and these patients therefore tend to be in the younger age-groups and are of employable age.

The suddenness of the accident and the psychological shock of losing an arm cannot be underestimated. The physiotherapist can do much to help the patient in this respect as she will be treating the patient from the day following the operation, and much will need to be done to prepare the patient for wearing and using a prosthesis.

The aims of physiotherapy are as follows:

(*i*) to strengthen and mobilize the entire shoulder girdle;

(*ii*) to prevent contractures;

(*iii*) to strengthen the muscles controlling the stump and maintain full range of movement in the joints;

(*iv*) to control oedema of the stump; and

(*v*) to maintain a good posture.

On the day following amputation, exercises to the shoulder girdle and unaffected arm are commenced. The patient will depend upon good mobility of this region for the control of his prosthesis.

The stump must remain in a good position and this must be supervised by both nurses and physiotherapists. The contracture most likely to develop in the above-elbow amputee is one of flexion, adduction and medial rotation at the shoulder, and frequently there is the danger of a frozen shoulder developing. The contracture most likely to occur in the below-elbow amputee is that of flexion at the elbow.

A few days following amputation, active exercises for the muscles controlling the stump can be started and gradually progressed to strong resisted exercises when the sutures are removed.

After the sutures are removed on the fourteenth day, firm stump bandaging is commenced in the same way and for the same reasons as for the lower limb amputee (see p. 302). A 3 inch (75 mm) wide 'Elset' or crepe bandage is used.

A constant check on the posture of the patient is necessary to ensure a level shoulder girdle and good position of the head and neck.

Four to five days postoperatively, a leather gauntlet can be applied over the bandage. Into this gauntlet simple tools such as cutlery in below-elbow stumps or a pencil or paintbrush can be fixed, and the patient encouraged to use his stump. Where possible early use of the stump for functional activities diminishes the risk of the patient becoming 'one-handed'.

Prosthetic stage

As soon as the sutures are removed the patient is seen by the Medical Officer, at the regional Limb Fitting Centre, and measurements are taken for a prosthesis.

At present it is not possible to fit the patient with a temporary prosthesis as in the case of the lower limb amputee, and the patient must wait two to three months for the manufacture of his definitive prosthesis. Sometimes at this stage the patient will be given a discarded 'second-hand' prosthesis of which the appropriate parts including the socket are remade, and arm training with this temporary prosthesis is commenced at the Limb Fitting Centre.

Usually the arm training units in the Limb Fitting Centres are staffed by occupational therapists, emphasis obviously being placed upon independence and training in functional skills and work and recreational activities.

A patient can be fitted with a heavy working arm, a light working arm or a dress arm which is purely a cosmetic prosthesis. In the first two cases, control of the prosthesis and of the terminal device is by straps which pass posteriorly across the patient's scapular region and which are activated by protraction of the scapula and extension of the stump (see Plate 12/15).

Numerous terminal devices are available, but all patients will be given a split hook (see Plates 12/16, 12/17) which can be used for many activities and is the most commonly used device, and a cosmetic hand. The occupational therapist will assess the patient and depending upon his work and hobbies he will be supplied with the relevant devices.

It is essential that the patient return to work or be trained for alternative employment as soon as possible, and normally these patients, once over the initial shock, are well motivated to do so.

BIBLIOGRAPHY

Anderson, M. H. *et al. Clinical Prosthetics for Physicians and Therapists.* Charles C. Thomas, Springfield, Ill., 1959.

Gillespie, J. A. (ed.). *Modern Trends in Vascular Surgery,* Vol. I. Butterworth, 1970.

Humm, W. *Rehabilitation of the Lower Limb Amputee.* Baillière Tindall, 2nd ed. 1969.

Klopsteg, P. E. and Wilson, P. D. *Human Limbs and their Substitutes.* Hafner Publishing Co., New York, 1969.

Murdoch, G. (ed.). *Prosthetic and Orthotic Practice.* Edward Arnold, 1970.

'Symposium on Limb Ablation and Limb Replacement', in *Annals of the Royal College of Surgeons of England,* April 1967, Vol. 40 No. 4.

Index